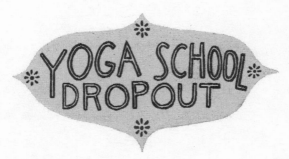

LUCY EDGE

EBURY
PRESS

First published in Great Britain in 2005

10 9 8 7 6 5 4

Text © Lucy Edge 2005

First published by
Ebury Press
Random House, 20 Vauxhall Bridge Road, London SW1V 2SA

Random House Australia (Pty) Limited
20 Alfred Street, Milsons Point, Sydney, New South Wales 2061, Australia

Random House New Zealand Limited
18 Poland Road, Glenfield, Auckland 10, New Zealand

Random House South Africa (Pty) Limited
Endulini, 5A Jubilee Road, Parktown 2193, South Africa

The Random House Group Limited Reg. No. 954009

www.randomhouse.co.uk

A CIP catalogue record for this book is available from the British Library.

Cover design by Two Associates
Text design and typesetting by seagulls
Cover illustration by David Dean

ISBN 0091899222

Papers used by Ebury Press are natural, recyclable products made from wood grown in sustainable forests.

Printed and bound in Great Britain by Mackays of Chatham plc

Contents

Chapter One

'The violet vibrations blow my crown chakra wide open' 1

Chapter Two

'Merging with the pool of cosmic bliss that is the universe' 9

Chapter Three

'Please be tucking in at all times' 27

Chapter Four

'Possessing only what is necessary' 51

Chapter Five

'Much sex is coming, much money is coming' 65

Chapter Six

'I need to be with gentle people' 95

Chapter Seven
'Durga, Durga, Durga' 111

Chapter Eight
'Get juicy' 125

Chapter Nine
'Stretch out upper eyelashes' 157

Chapter Ten
'An ocean of love' 185

Chapter Eleven
'A hump is there, like a camel' 205

Chapter Twelve
'My kleshas really fucked me' 235

Chapter Thirteen
'Not all nine hundred and ninety-nine holes are plugged at once' 253

Chapter Fourteen
'That's one big-ass crystal' 269

Chapter Fifteen
'Atcha! OM! Boom!' 297

Recipe for Apple Muffins 315
Glossary 317
Useful Contacts 331
Further Reading 337
Permissions 339
Thanks 341

For Mum and Dad – my first gurus,
and for Teddy Edge – my two-year-old godson and guru-in-chief

I have used the real names and identities of the gurus, yoga teachers, ashrams and schools, but to protect the innocent people I met along the way I have changed some names and details. The description of a career in advertising is a melding of many experiences and not representative of any one particular agency.

~ 1 ~

'The violet vibrations blow my crown chakra wide open'

'Yoga student!' said the rickshaw driver, nodding emphatically in the direction of a bungalow just visible in the fading light, beyond the orange flowers of several flamboyant canna plants.

'Two hundred rupees! You pay!' he said, even more emphatically, stopping just short of a grumpy cow, which was occupying most of the narrow road.

This was around £2.50 – a bit steep for a journey of half a mile in India – but if it delivered me to Ortario and Magdali's Café, reputedly the centre of Mysore yoga student life, well, it would be worth it. I'd only arrived in town an hour ago but I was desperate to start getting to know my yogic soulmates, and I was hungry.

I handed over the money and, after some delicate negotiations with a goat that was trying to make a meal of a poster on the gate, I headed up the garden path towards a long, messy row of beaten-up Birkenstocks. I added my shiny new orange Birkies to the line, took a deep breath and opened the door to yoga heaven.

There before me were twenty or more beautiful people, draped over floor cushions, daybeds and each other. A harassed waiter, the only person showing any signs of movement, shuttled backwards and forwards through shuttered kitchen doors from which the smell of garlic and fresh coriander periodically escaped.

Smiling weakly, I surveyed the scene, nervously clutching my brand new copy of *The Yoga Sutras of Patanjali* to my chest. I suddenly felt overwhelmed. I had imagined this moment for a long time – my first encounter with the yoga students of Mysore – but where to sit? Everyone seemed so entwined. Unable to work out an immediate way to add myself to this human spaghetti, I hovered at the edge of a small splinter group sitting straight-backed at a low-slung table decorated with empty plates, bits of Naan bread and mint tea.

'Would you like to join us?' asked a husky-voiced girl with golden skin and long, white-blonde hair.

'Thank you, I'd love to,' I said gratefully.

I attempted to copy their 'lotus' position – ankles perched effort-lessly on their thighs – but my hips and knees resisted at the crucial 45-degree point. I was forced to abandon the attempt and sit cross-legged – feet and ankles nailed firmly to the ground. I slid my shawl over the offending posture.

'I'm Lisa, from Sweden,' said the blonde girl, with a perfect English accent and a warm smile.

'I'm Lucy. I just arrived today, from London.'

'*Namaste*, Lucy. Welcome to Mysore.' Lisa raised her hands into prayer position and bowed her head. 'This is Greg, and Shanti.'

'*Namaste*,' said Greg, pressing his palms into prayer position and bowing his head.

'*Namaste*,' said Shanti, doing the same.

'*Namaste*,' I replied, bowing in return and thus completing our round of promises that the spirit in each of us would respect the spirit in each other.

I was eager to find out more about these fellow spirits.

'I love your outfit, Shanti,' I said, admiring the tiger-eye browns and yellows of the *salwar kameez* that perfectly offset her mahogany corkscrew curls, olive skin and translucent green eyes.

'Oh, thank you. Actually it's very old; my yoga teacher's wife gave it to me. Isn't that so sweet? She's so beautiful.'

Warming to my subject, I added, 'And your shawl – where did you get it? It's such a great colour on you.'

'Oh, thank you so much, Lucy. You know what, before I came here I was in Dharamshala and this holy man read my aura – the shawl was a perfect match. The violet vibrations blow my crown *chakra* wide open, but it also keeps my energy field protected. The gold trim – see here,' Shanti showed us the intricate embroidery, 'helps my spirit guides look out for me.'

'Your shawl is pretty too, Lucy,' said Lisa kindly.

'Oh, thank you. St Joseph of Brompton Cross. It was expensive, about two hundred pounds, I think, but on a cost-per-wear basis it's actually worked out to be a bit of a bargain.'

A small gap seemed to have opened up in the conversation.

Lisa came to my rescue. 'What brought you to India, Lucy?'

'I think it was a Boeing seven-four-seven. It was a long journey – into Bombay and then on to Bangalore. I'm feeling pretty awful now but that might be more to do with how much I had to drink on the plane than jet lag.'

There was another gap in the conversation; it seemed a little larger than the last.

Lisa smiled indulgently. 'What about you, Shanti?'

'I am here to study *Ashtanga* with Guruji. I told you earlier, before Lucy arrived, that it was my first time in Mysore but actually I've been to the city before – I just don't remember it. My mom was here in seventy-five when she was pregnant with me – she didn't know she was pregnant so she was doing all these inversions – *adho mukha vrksasana, parsva pada sarvangasana, hanumanasana* in *sirsasana*. Pretty dangerous really – she coulda lost me – but I must have loved it. It feels like yoga is in my blood.'

'Your mum must have been one of the Guruji's first Western students,' said Lisa admiringly.

Shanti smiled in acquiescence and, with a dancer's poise, slowly unfurled her legs into an easy 180-degree stretch, keeping her back perfectly straight. She flexed her ankles and toes and came to rest with a small tinkle of the hand-carved bells on her antique ankle chains.

Greg, a pale-faced, skinny man with a thin ponytail and a goatee plaited with yellow thread, watched appreciatively. He cleared his throat. 'My father spent some time in India back then – actually it was even earlier – sixty-eight, I think. He was on a rescue mission to bring home my *chillum*-soaked aunt. She'd been hanging out with the Beatles in Rishikesh at Maharishi Mahesh Yogi's ashram. I went to stay with her when she got back home to Woodstock, I wanted her to teach me how to fly over people's heads like the Maharishi but she said I was too young so she taught me some yoga instead. That experience really rocked my world. I was on my path. Yogaaahhh,' he breathed, spreading his palms wide as if to embrace the world. He smiled beatifically, especially at Shanti.

Lisa bubbled enthusiastically, 'I love that we all came to yoga at such a young age. I was given *The Yoga Sutras of Patanjali* when I was thirteen by my older sister. I remember reading it in our summerhouse in Gotland. It was a real turning point for me – a spiritual epiphany. They say that we choose the family that we are born into. It seems,' she beamed, 'that we all chose well.'

Greg and Shanti smiled in agreement. My smile was a little weaker. My favourite reading material at thirteen was *Jackie* magazine; when the

Beatles and Greg's aunt had discovered Maharishi Mahesh Yogi, my father had been working his arse off to buy us a colour telly; I'd worked in advertising all of my adult life, and the only spiritual epiphany I had ever experienced had been at the bottom of a bottle of Pinot Grigio. I quickly changed the subject – was Shanti a yoga teacher? I thought it likely.

Shanti's diamond nose stud glinted in the fading light. 'Oh yeah, of course. I've been a teacher for eight years. I started by helping my mom with her students. Now I teach privately all over Manhattan, and in Brooklyn, where I live. I have twenty regular students and a website – you can buy my first DVD on it. It's a great flow, I think you'd love it. I'm not pushing it too hard – it's kinda organic. I'm letting it grow naturally.' She fished around in her large mirrored bag and pulled out some business cards. 'Here, take one each – it has my website address. Let me know what y'all think of the DVD.'

We thanked her profusely, admiring the thin creamy cards on which *Lakshmi*, goddess of wealth and prosperity, was depicted in a pink sari and golden headdress, standing in a lotus flower, gold coins pouring forth from one of her four hands.

Greg hurried to give us his business cards, which carried a golden embossed OM, and to tell us that he was studying with Guruji, was also a yoga teacher back home and lived in Brooklyn too, just like Shanti. He described his work as a *Raso Vai* massage therapist with mounting excitement: 'I walk up and down the body, using hot oil to bring energy flow and harmony to the joints. It's an amazing spiritual experience. I invite bliss, love and higher consciousness to pour through me to you,' he said, his gaze fixed on the clear object of his affection.

Shanti smiled and, with her legs still at 180 degrees, lazily stretched her body out so that her torso lay completely flat to the floor, her face resting comfortably in her hands.

'Have you ever slipped?' I asked.

He gave me a stern look. 'I may be heavy with the weight of my spiritual duty, Lucy, but I'm pretty light on my feet, plus I use a rope to steady myself.' He got up. 'I've gotta get my beauty sleep – I'm on my mat at five tomorrow morning and I'm hoping Guruji is going to give me some help with my drop backs.' He gave Shanti one more longing look and loped off into the night.

Shanti slowly raised herself off the floor and languidly rotated her body, bending over one of her outstretched legs so that her head touched her ankle. She raised her head just a couple of inches to tell us that she was starting tomorrow morning at six o'clock. This would be a lie-in as she normally got up at four every day, except Sundays and moon days. She wrapped her hands around her foot and slowly returned her head to her ankle.

Lisa loved getting up early, too. 'My five a.m. practice is so right for me. It's such a *sattvic*, pure, harmonious time of day – my mind is clear and my body feels amazing afterwards, so serene.'

I decided not to mention that I was hoping to be on my mat no earlier than nine in the morning but I did have to make one confession: that I wasn't studying with Guruji.

Shanti raised her head from her ankle and stared at me. There was silence.

Sensing that this gap in the conversation was about to turn itself into a yawning chasm, I rushed to explain myself. 'It's just that I did a workshop with Guruji in London and he called me a "bad lady". I had a collapsing crocodile, you know, the press-up position.'

'*Chaturanga dandasana,*' corrected Shanti.

'Then he tried to get me into that balancing position involving standing on one leg and taking hold of the big toe of the other foot.'

'*Utthita hasta padangusthasana,*' said Shanti, helpfully.

Explaining that I'd lost my balance and nearly toppled him and had therefore thought it best to start my studies in India with someone else, I quickly moved on to describe the six-week course that I had signed up for with Mr Venkatesh. 'He is the author of his own system of yoga – "*Atma Vikasa*" – it means "evolution of the soul",' I added proudly.

'Ah Venkatesh – the so-called "Rubber Yogi".' Lisa looked down at my crossed legs (the shawl had slipped off) with a doubtful expression.

For the third time in half an hour I smiled weakly.

Somehow I'd lost my appetite.

~2~

'Merging with the pool of cosmic bliss that is the universe'

The fact that I was struggling to feel at home in Mysore was hardly surprising. Only one week before I had added my shiny orange Birkies to the line-up outside Ortario and Magdali's Café, I had been striding down the ad agency corridors in high heels, on my way to a meeting about a tub of margarine. Spending more than a decade in advertising debating the meaning of such tubs hadn't been ideal preparation for a yoga student in search of life's deeper meaning:

'Talk to me about polyunsaturated fat, Lucy,' said the Creative Director as he pulled me onto his knee.

I was uncomfortable with this subtle shift in power but I couldn't work out how to slide off without causing a scene. As my toes searched quietly but desperately for the ground, I explained the latest strategic problem facing our beleaguered margarine client:

'Polyunsaturated fat has, until now, been seen by the consumer as good fat, but monounsaturated fat is even better – it's the next big thing. Our client plans to launch one next month but it's likely that Sainsbury's and Tesco's will follow. The client is worried because people think that a supermarket's own brand is basically the same product as the more expensive brands and don't want to pay the extra.'

I used the Creative Director's momentary lapse in concentration to slide further off his knee. Aahh. Getting there slowly, one toe firmly on the floor. I continued steadily:

'So we need to give our monounsaturated fat an emotional advantage – something that will differentiate it from own label. The client wants to use his existing advertising equity – the sunflowers – because research says they have happy and carefree values, particularly if they sing happy, care-free songs. The problem is that the sunflowers also say polyunsaturated. So the question is – do we use the sunflowers and risk consumer confusion? And if we do use them, then what the heck song are they going to sing?'

The Creative Director tightened his grip around my waist and smirked. 'I love it when you talk dirty, Lucy.'

You can see the problem.

We worked seventy-hour weeks to answer these questions. This would have been understandable if we had been creating world peace, but deciding what sunflowers should sing shouldn't have kept us in the office so long.

There were some odd moments of relief – wearing pink fluffy Agent Provocateur mules in imitation of a domestic goddess for a vacuum cleaner pitch, sporting a purple, crushed-velvet Pussy Galore mini-skirt and thigh-length boots to sing 'Happy Birthday' to my marge client, to name but two. But somehow these compensations were not enough. I was fed up with working at the centre of the periphery. Surely there was more to life?

All of this talk about marge left little time for a private life. An M&S Café Culture ready meal, especially the Aubergine Parmigiana, became an icon of domestic bliss. There was no time to go out and play, only time to stay in and recover before the next deadline came flying across my desk like a cruise missile. Guaranteed to seek, find and destroy all chance of finding a man before I hit the retirement home.

I tried to look on my almost permanent single status positively – no need to have more than one set of good underwear, no beer taking up fridge space that would be better devoted to Diet Coke, M&S chocolate peanuts and Pinot Grigio, none of the pain of intimate waxing, no fights over the remote control, no left-up loo seats – but it was clear that I would rather have a man than these advantages.

The few relationships I did have were disasters.

A vintage art director in vintage black leather coat and vintage Porsche took me to the Notting Hill restaurant 192 and said: 'Lucy, you are very special, an extraordinary woman.' He was clearly so over-whelmed by my extraordinariness that he couldn't pick up the phone to arrange another date.

A very promising young copywriter kissed me in a jazz club at 3 a.m. We exchanged emails the next day:

From: Lucy Edge
To: A Very Promising Young Copywriter

Thanks for a great night. I've never been to Ronnie Scott's before but now I'm going to go all the time. Your session on the sax was wonderful – I felt the room fall away, as if you were playing just for me. Can't wait to see you again. I'd love to go out on your boat as discussed. How about Thursday next week? Think I can swing it – I can pretend I'm in Sheffield talking to ladies about marge. x

From: A Very Promising Young Copywriter
To: Lucy Edge

It was a great night – loved every minute of it. Babe, I meant everything I said then – you're great, you really are – but today is another day and I think we should move on. Might be best to give the boat a miss just till things calm down, huh? Would you be a darling and bring me some more of those facts about sunflowers that you were telling me last night? Don't seem to be able to recall the finer details and I know they would make for some great copy. Want to make sure I can add Yellow Pencil to the awards shelf this year. Thanks Babe. x

Not to be deterred, I went to Paris with another copywriter, a divorcing Catholic who was so terrified of his soon-to-be ex-wife finding out that he had been away for the weekend with another woman that he stuffed £300 in my jacket pocket as we picked up our baggage at Charles de Gaulle, 'to cover expenses'.

He announced on the plane home: 'You know, Lucy, this weekend; it's not been a cold thing. I like you more than I thought I would but I'm not ready for any commitment at the moment. You could be Cameron Diaz and I'd feel the same way.'

Six months later he was re-married, and her name wasn't Cameron. I should have demanded more cash.

At best, I thought, I was a Canapé Girl, a bite-sized morsel that kept a man going before he met The One. At worst I was little more than a hooker working the baggage reclaim carousel.

I tried employing the analytical skills I used as an advertising planner to work out what had gone wrong each time, but I always ended up having to convene summit meetings with my girlfriends – the 'Cappuccino Gurus'. We would run through the options over coffee and biscotti in Café Violette or Café Seventy-Nine. Perhaps he thought I wasn't interested? Perhaps he just wasn't interested enough? Perhaps he was a commitment phobe? Perhaps it was me that was the commitment phobe? Was I emotionally autistic or was it him? There were many theories but in the end there was only one inescapable conclusion: in all of these messed-up relationships there was one common denominator, and that was me.

Clearly I needed to make some changes, to find a different way of seeing the world and living in it, to discover a more balanced, less isolated way of life.

What were the options? With the exception of Café Culture ready meals and the Cappuccino Gurus, the only things that had really sustained me during The Advertising Years were Joseph, Pinot Grigio, yoga and my mum. I had found some answers to life's biggest questions in the bottom of a bottle several times but, sadly, had woken up in the morning unable to recall exactly what they were. My mum always thought she had the answer but sometimes I disagreed. And even I, after years of trying, had to concede that lasting happiness probably didn't lie in another pretty dress.

That left yoga.

I had always been impressed by my friend Maria's party trick – picking up a pack of Kellogg's Corn Flakes between her buttocks as she performed the splits. She attributed this feat to a strict regime of *Iyengar* yoga, which apparently involved blocks, bolsters and standing on your head for ten minutes. I wasn't sure how this helped open your groin, and anyway I wasn't tempted. It took the end of another relationship and a recuperative holiday in Tobago to get me to my first yoga class.

I met tiny, gorgeous Kate on that holiday in Tobago, in 1997. She was travelling alone, her only company a blue, sticky mat and yoga practice tape recorded by her London teacher. She spent the afternoons basking by the pool in a yellow bikini and baseball hat, quietly reading the three-inch-thick Paramahansa Yogananda's *Autobiography of a Yogi*, and the early evenings on the hotel lawn making every single one of twenty different *asana* (yoga postures) look effortless, as if they had come floating down from heaven on the wings of angels. I noticed that her bendy, pretzel-like body and graceful, soft yogic actions left her looking at peace with the world and cast an unearthly spell over the male guests – they ordered endless rum punches just to remain in her vicinity, and sat mesmerized, unable to speak, or move. By the end of the holiday she had a boyfriend, and I had the name of her teacher: Simon Low.

I rang him the following week. Simon told me that he was taking a group to Huzur Vadisi in south-west Turkey in two weeks' time. The group would be of mixed ability and it was fine that I was a complete beginner. I read the brochure over and over again. We would practise yoga under a canopy of grapes, in a valley surrounded by pine forest. Our afternoons would be spent sunbathing by the stone swimming pool or dozing in shady hammocks, listening to cicadas. In the evenings we would play chess and read ancient Urdu poetry in the wooden *kosk*, an overgrown tree house. We would sleep in nomadic *yurts*, circular domed tents with a hole in the roof, the 'eye of heaven', built for stargazing.

I could hardly wait. In less than a month I would have a pretzel-like body, and all of its incumbent powers.

Needless to say, things didn't work out exactly as planned.

While the rest of the class, many of whom had been doing yoga for ten years or more, focused on lengthening their muscles and dropping into the pose – 'relaxing into it, like warm, gloopy custard' – I concentrated on not falling over. I wobbled my way through the week, shaking uncontrollably as my muscles released years of tension.

I was permanently out of sync with my fellow students. It reminded me of the early days of learning step aerobics in the gym – when my arms and legs stubbornly resisted any attempt to move in the same direction as everyone else. I always spoilt the beautiful symmetrical line that would otherwise have been created by twenty pink g-string leotards moving in perfect synchronicity. Just when I'd worked out what Simon was asking me to do, and attempted to do it, everyone else was onto the next thing.

I learned that *asana* can help us change old patterns established in the body and, when combined with regulated breathing practices, or *pranayama*, and some meditation, could start to unite the mind, body and breath. So much for the theory … Simon's intonations were unusually buttery, his voice was soft and rich, like shortbread dipped in honey, but it was all in vain. When he asked me to inhale and open myself to new experiences, I exhaled. When he asked me to exhale and let go of the past, I held my breath, leaving my personal history locked firmly within.

The only time I did manage any degree of synchronicity was poolside. In the daily sunbathing line-up I found co-coordinating the laying down of my beach towel alongside those of others almost effortless.

Meanwhile, back on the yoga mat, my troubles continued. My hamstrings shouted from the rooftops, opening my hips was like trying to open a door whose hinges had been painted over twenty times in as many years and I couldn't persuade my shoulders to end their life-long love affair with my ears. I couldn't even stand up straight. If I held my tummy in I couldn't breathe, if I pushed out my chest my bottom stuck out, if I pulled up my kneecaps my calf muscles tightened. Far from being able to stand on my head or my hands, by the end of class I couldn't even stand on my own two feet.

Try as I might, I couldn't create enough yogic fire to raise the *kundalini* serpent of energy from the bottom of my spine, every single one of my *chakras* remained resolutely closed for business, and I couldn't count more than three breaths without thinking about what was for dinner. It seemed unlikely that I would be following Simon's instruction to merge the energies of *ha* (the hot energy of the sun) and *tha* (the cool energy of the moon) into my *sushumna* (the energy channel running up the centre of the spine) at any time in the near future.

Kate had told me that *The Bhagavad Gita* – 'The Lord's Song', the ancient scripture – says people only come to practise yoga in this life if they have already practised it in a previous life. If this was the case, my body had forgotten all about it. I could only be grateful that yoga wasn't conducted in teams – I would never have been picked. It wasn't just the lack of co-ordination and flexibility; there was also the complete absence of muscle definition and stamina. I had never been 'good at games'.

I finished each class completely exhausted, shaking and not quite myself until I had sat by the pool in the afternoon sun for five hours. People tried not to look alarmed but I could tell they were exchanging worried looks and had agreed a covert mission of keeping a watchful eye on me at all times. They tried to comfort me with tales of how long it had taken them to be able to touch their toes but I could tell, even at this early stage, that my ticket to yoga heaven wasn't stamped 'Fast-Track'.

Simon gently explained to the few beginners in the group, as we tried to relax our aching muscles amongst the cushions in the wooden *kosk*, that yoga is one of six strands of Hindu *darshana* or 'ways of seeing', that it can help us 'peel back the layers, like the layers of an onion', enabling us to see ourselves more clearly and 'awakening us to new possibilities, new ways of being'. Yoga would help us find deep within our core, hidden away like buried treasure, nothing less than our true Self – a changeless, stable, quiet Self, sometimes called the 'Eternal Self' – quite distinct from the highly flammable, ever-changing emotions, mind and body with which we misidentify ourselves.

Yoga would reveal this Eternal Self by a process known as *chitta vritti nirodhah* – 'the control of the activities of the mind'. This control wouldn't be about repression of thoughts and closing down, but about being aware, observing these activities, developing the skills to remove the roadblock of mental chatter that stands in the way of inner stillness. If we practised regularly, Simon told us, 'our mind would remain calm, peaceful and clear-sighted, whatever the situation', 'enabling us to meet life and all of its challenges head-on'. Yes, even the mosquitoes that dive-bombed our mats would be met with equanimity.

It was a difficult week – as befits the peeling of an onion I shed quite a lot of tears – but miraculously, given my struggles on the mat, there were glimpses of a rare calm; my mind, breath and body seemed to be getting along and the mental whirlings – the *chitta vritti* – did occasionally stop for a second or two. I was so stiff I had to ask for help getting out of bed in the morning, but beneath the rigor mortis were some encouraging signs of muscle growth and every last drop of tension had been squeezed out of me, which must have been really weighing me down because I lost four pounds. I have a photograph of Simon and me at the end of the holiday – he is smiling, tanned and relaxed, strong and centred in his sarong and Prana vest; I look knackered and a bit wobbly, but I also look happy, and it wasn't just the weight loss. Beyond the smile on my face I could feel my body beginning to smile – a big smile of relief – as it let go of all those tensions.

And there was something else – a feeling that somehow something fundamental had shifted, as Simon had said, an opening up to other possibilities. I told my *yurt*mate, Caroline, a ladylike reality TV producer with a swinging blonde bob, about this feeling – this awareness of something beyond my yoga mat that I couldn't quite name – as we lay beneath the stars sharing a spliff. She thought that this glimmer of awareness might be a glimpse of *samadhi*, of enlightenment itself.

Caroline told me that when we eventually found the Eternal Self we would go beyond the demands of our ego, beyond what we own and what we want. Our feelings of separateness, our sense of difference from others would disappear and we would rest in the Self-Realized state of *samadhi* – a state of sublime peace, of enlightenment. She assured me: 'We won't worry about men or our appearance or our job, or even the mosquitoes, because we will be merging with the pool of cosmic bliss that is the universe. In this cosmic consciousness we will be in touch with all of existence, with a world beyond thought, a liberated world of infinite love, free from all suffering, in perfect harmony with ourselves and each other.'

I did have a spot of bother getting to grips with this idea until I'd had a few more spliffs – at which point merging with the big pool of cosmic bliss that is the universe suddenly became as easy as lying by the pool.

Back home in London, my tan down the plughole, the noise of traffic outside my door and my bikini in the washing machine, I lost any glimmer of cosmic certainty but I made some headway with the continuing battle to unite breath and body, if not mind.

In my now thrice-weekly yoga classes, I stopped wobbling when both my feet were still firmly on the ground, reserving feelings of unsteadiness for those times I was clutching a foot to my forehead. I touched my toes for the first time in my adult life (day 366). I lay down on the ground and got my feet to touch the floor behind my head in *halasana* or 'plough' (day 872). I got stronger and managed to stay in poses for more than one breath before collapsing on my mat. My stamina improved so that I was able to make it to the end of the class without needing to spend half of it resting on my knees, head to the ground, in 'child's pose' – though it remains to this day my favourite pose. Even my co-ordination improved; I knew I would never make it as a synchronised swimmer but I was no longer an embarrassment to myself, or the rest of the class. I felt more balanced and could stand on one leg for at least ten seconds before I fell over and occasionally I caught a glimpse, in the far distance, of some much-needed equilibrium.

Unfortunately, these glimpses were rare and stilling the activities of my mind presented a continuing challenge. Resting in *savasana* or 'corpse pose' at the end of class, I was a heaving mass of *chitta vritti*. Was the handsome man on the next mat single? Should I try to make conversation as we put our yoga mats away? Would anyone want to go for a glass of wine after class?

The answer to this last question was always yes, and it normally turned into more than one glass. By the time we hit the second bottle my classmates were freely admitting the contents of their *chitta vritti*. It wasn't always about the person on the next mat. *Chitta vritti* could also concern what to wear to a party, whether to ask the boss for a raise, what to have for dinner tomorrow night, or whether the iron had been left on. These were the thoughts that stood between us and cosmic bliss.

Several years passed. My classmates went on yoga world tours and came back with lofty ideals: giving up their high-powered jobs in favour of running yoga centres, or becoming yoga teachers and selling yoga clothes made from organic Peruvian cotton. They told me stories of 'deepening their practice' under the strict tutelage of exotic-sounding gurus – T.K.V. Desikachar, Pattabhi Jois (known, I discovered later, as 'Guruji') and B.K.S. Iyengar. The schools didn't sound as glamorous as those of London – instead of fluffy white towels, incense sticks and candles there were concrete floors and bars on the windows. Elasticated-waist trousers and baggy T-shirts replaced Nuala and Prana yoga clothes, certainly as far as Desikachar and Iyengar were concerned. But no matter – these schools got results. Caroline told us that she'd had a spiritual epiphany whilst cleaning the toilet at the Sivananda Ashram, a 12-acre 'Garden of Eden' in Kerala. Jim and Jessie, who had also been on that Turkish holiday, had met a girl who'd been to the Bihar School of Yoga where she'd worn white pyjamas, surrendered her passport and shaved her head as a symbol of her lack of ego and worldly thoughts.

Shaven heads notwithstanding, my fascination with the 5,000-year-old traditions of yoga grew. I began to have dreams about going to India. This land of mountains and sages. This land of shrines and saints. This land in which everything – the air, the trees, the ground you walked on – could apparently help you find yourself, and cosmic bliss.

Paramahansa Yogananda's *Autobiography of a Yogi*, the book Kate was reading in Tobago, was peppered with stories of masters equipped with extraordinary powers over matter. Vishudhananda – 'The Perfume Saint' – could rearrange the structure of 'lifetrons', particles smaller than atoms, to create whatever perfume or piece of fruit you desired. 'The Tiger Swami' used his mind power to focus energy and had a bet with the Prince of Cooch Behar that he could use his bare hands to resist and bind the newly caught tiger Raja Begum and depart the tiger's cage in a conscious manner. He won the bet and trumped it by putting his head in the mouth of the tiger, although he did then spend six months in bed with blood poisoning as the enraged tiger had dug his claws in at this piece of effrontery. Then there was Swami Pranabanada, 'The Saint with Two Bodies', who could talk to a friend on the shores of the Ganges at the same time as he spoke to the twelve-year-old Paramahansa Yogananda at home.

I wished that I could be 'The Ad Girl with Two Bodies' – leaving one of me to earn good money for talking about marge while the other me went off to have adventures with these masters.

Yoga became the perfect antidote to the demands of life in advertising. My expenditure on Triyoga and Life Centre classes, Nuala tank tops and Calmia Meditation Mist began to outstrip the amount spent in Joseph, but I felt that I had to keep this growing attachment to myself. One of the Account Directors, on seeing a note pinned to my desk with Gandhi's words 'We must be the change in the world we want to see', looked at me suspiciously and took me out for lunch. He told me, over his duck on a bed of green lentils, that he didn't think yoga and a career in advertising were really compatible – his girlfriend came home from yoga class rather spaced-out, and with some strange notions concerning a merger with cosmic bliss. I got the message.

I started to lead a double life. A week at Ibiza Yoga was cunningly disguised as a week of heavy clubbing action. If I came into the office stiff from a particularly gruelling class I would blame my walk on muscles pickled in alcohol. Sometimes they actually were so I wasn't lying all the time.

I would probably still be leading this double life were it not for the final straw. I woke up one day to find myself the victim of a power coup.

It was time to move on.

Leaving the singing sunflowers to make their own way in the world, I would follow in my friends' footsteps and escape to India. I would take a six-month career break and go on a yoga school pilgrimage.

I would find a guru, someone to lead me from *gu*, darkness, to *ru*, light. Someone to help me unite body, breath and mind, and strip away the layers of ego. He would direct me in my search for deeper meaning, a fulfilling way of life. He would help me find my purpose, my place in the world. Perhaps that place would be up a mountain – where I would, like others before me, merge my Eternal Self with the big pool of cosmic bliss that is the universe.

In my dreams I returned a Yoga Goddess, the embodiment of feminine perfection – peaceful, happy, loving, wise, endlessly compassionate towards a suffering world – and a magnetic babe attracting strong and sweaty, yet emotionally vulnerable men. We would share profound moments, wrapped in hammocks debating the teachings of *The Bhagavad Gita*, the spiritual struggle of the human soul.

In my dreams not only had my purpose in life been revealed but also a pretzel-like body – light on fat, flexible yet strong. I would sit in the lotus position, or stand on my head, effortlessly performing advanced postures in designer clothes for a *Sunday Telegraph* feature on Yoga Babes. *Vogue* would photograph me in my favourite organic juice bar and designer friends would choose me to model their size eight scented knickers. In these dreams the lack of money didn't matter because I was beyond materialism, and anyway I got free holidays when Sting invited me to his Italian villa to give him personal tuition.

Of course, in discussion with the Cappuccino Gurus, I recognized that it might not turn out this way, but it had to be better than another winter of late-night ready meals for one in front of the telly.

I decided to approach the yoga school selection process in the same way I worked through complex strategic problems in advertising – with methodical research. I went to W.H. Smith and bought a pink file and ten plastic wallets.

There was a bewildering array of yogic paths. Which way to go? It was very confusing. The royal and scientific path of *Raja* yoga with Desikachar in Chennai? The path of self-knowledge – *Jnana* yoga – at Tiruvannamalai? *Bhakti* yoga – the path of love and devotion – with a Hugging Mother on the Keralan backwaters? Sri Aurobindo's *Integral* yoga at Auroville? *Tantra* – worshipping the body as a temple of the Divine – with Osho in Pune? The precision of *Iyengar* yoga, also in Pune? *Ashtanga* in Mysore or *Sivananda* in Kerala? These places occupied the four corners of India – should I go north, south, east or west?

I decided to take the Pink File, by now so fat with yogic possibility that I could hardly close it, on a yoga holiday in the south of France, where I could mull things over.

The villa was home to the bohemian Ted and Cat, sculptor and muse. During the summer they lived in Ted's studio and rented out the cool, shuttered bedrooms of their farmhouse. They spent lunchtime on their terrace and, after a couple of jugs of lesser-known Luberon wine, they would move to Ted's studio. I think this was the time when Cat fulfilled her role as Ted's muse most effectively – I could hear his gratitude from my place by the pool.

Lying there late one steamy afternoon, trying not to listen to Cat inspiring Ted, I got talking to fellow holidaymaker Richard. He had just resigned from his job as a call centre manager in Plymouth and, like me, was planning to travel around the yoga schools of India.

We lay by day under Ted and Cat's fig trees and contemplated our future beyond the fields of lavender and thyme. In fact, I was contemplating his strong arms and full swimming trunks, but I think I did it without him noticing. We mooched around the market buying tomatoes, Cavaillon melons and stoneground bread stuffed with olives. Our elbows touched. We shared spliffs and talk of yogic paths as we sat dangling our feet in the cool darkness of the 2 a.m. swimming pool.

'I've been to India several times, you know, babe,' said Richard, during one of these night-time conversations. 'Spent a year in the Himalaya when I was eighteen – wow. Almost rocked back home in orange robes – way too much *chillum*. But I learned some stuff when I was up the mountain. Had a *kundalini* experience, you know. Certainly woke up old Shakti the serpent. I could feel her blazing her way up my spine, unlocking all of my *chakras*, and then she met Shiva right up at the crown of my head. Wow, man, it was like an explosion, cosmic bliss. I was the universe and the universe was me. We were one. I was in love with the whole fucking world, man. Boom Shiva!'

Had Richard had direct experience of *samadhi*, the enlightened world that Caroline had described to me under the stars in Turkey? Or was he just a stone-head?

'Were you in India on your own?' I asked.

'I was alone in the Himalaya, just me and the crazy old guys together, smoking *chillum* and talking crazy stuff. I met a woman when I came down the mountain – at Osho's place in Pune. Have you heard of him? He's the so-called "Sex Guru".'

I had actually. Jim and Jessie had visited the resort for a few days and warned me that I'd need some maroon and some white robes if I wanted to visit, and to be careful about sitting beneath the resort's bamboo trees, as they'd heard that people were prone to having sex in these picturesque spots, though they hadn't seen it themselves. I had to admit to being intrigued but I wasn't sure sex in a public place, with or without robes, would be my kind of thing.

Richard explained that he thought the press had sensationalized Osho's message, suggesting that Osho believed in promiscuous sex, when what Osho had actually said was that sex can be a meditative experience but only if you have mastery over it, not if you are a slave to it. 'This older bird really helped me with understanding that. One night, it was like she was calling me. I got over to her room as fast as I could and there she was, in the darkness, sitting on the floor, naked except for a red scarf, waiting for me. I learned to control myself in those two days, you know, to achieve that mastery. I was arrested a couple of days later for having a kilo of weed in my bag. Boom Shiva! I had to give the police guy a huge bribe to get off. Left Pune sharpish after that.'

He looked at me intently. 'So babe, let's rock up in India together. It'll be mad.' Mad is what it will be, I thought. Ah well, whatever else, it would be an adventure.

'OK,' I said, dipping my toes hesitantly back in the water. It was cold and I shivered.

We arranged to leave England for Mysore on 17 November. We'd both heard about Mr Venkatesh and wanted to do his six-week Union course, and then we'd sail to the bone-white beaches of the remote Andaman and Nicobar Islands for a New Year mini-break.

Perhaps it would all work out. I allowed myself to dream. There were the two of us, wearing necklaces of shell and headbands of bark fibre in keeping with island tradition. We would practise early morning yoga on the beach, and afterwards we would swim – the slow pulse of the tropical waters a welcome respite for our tired muscles, achingly stretched into limbs of lean goldenness. Perhaps we would breathe in perfect synchronicity, our sunbeds shaded by the mangrove trees, side by side in perfect alignment, a pleasing mirror of our unified souls.

Perhaps not. The day before we were due to leave, Richard sent me an email. Unwelcome news:

To: Babe!
From: Richard

Babe! Broken boiler. Got to fix so I can rent out the flat. I'll only be a week. Tops. Promise.
Boom Shiva!
R x

There were other rumours circulating in my Yahoo Inbox – one of the Cappuccino Gurus informed me that he'd fallen for a cocktail waitress dancing on a nightclub podium. What to do? Carry on as planned, that's what.

~ 3 ~

'Please be tucking in at all times'

I bounced out of Bangalore in the back of a white Ambassador. The red leather seats were deeply ingrained with the smell of stale tobacco – as befits a car that has been ruling the roads of India since 1947. Initially I was alarmed by the prospect of travelling in a fifty-year-old vehicle but the man who had won the bitterly fought 'Battle of the Drivers' (involving a lot of shouting and wild arm movements) at Bangalore airport insisted that it had 'plenty of features, madam'. The suspension looked as if it had given up the ghost, but the feature that swung it for me was the large picture of Elvis, trimmed with gold tinsel, hanging from the rear-view mirror.

I was happy to get out of the city – it was too busy celebrating its status as the power behind the burgeoning Indian computer industry to welcome a newly arrived yoga student. A copy of *The Bangalore Times*, thoughtfully left by the car's previous inhabitant, carried photographs of happy partygoers wearing heavily embroidered saris, gold jewellery and the big, relaxed smiles of the newly rich. As we sat in traffic – the only thing that moves slowly in Bangalore – I caught glimpses of home entertainment shops bursting with handsome Indian men in Western clothes. They debated the various merits of one home cinema system over another as they smoked Dunhill cigarettes. I imagined them jumping into the shiny new Japanese cars parked outside, blasting out the latest Bollywood or Justin Timberlake hit as they drove past the huge billboards advertising Scotch whisky and designer clothes, towards their beautiful homes in the newly built gated communities.

Leaving the city required a fast adjustment from the noise and speed of a twenty-first-century technology heaven to centuries-old quiet roads, lined with tattered palm trees. We passed women carrying the entire contents of fields on their heads, oxen pulling carts laboriously down the centre of the road and coconut-sellers using such large knives to slice off the top of the coconut that if they'd made a mistake they would surely have lost their entire arm.

I had imagined that sandalwood, Mysore's trademark scent, would come wafting down the approach road to greet me as we entered the city. There would be peaceful, shady, tree-lined avenues arranged around squares filled with statues of Gandhi and many benches from which to observe fountains exuberant with civic spirit. Women in this season's pink would lovingly tend cheeky-monkey children as they played with wooden toys. Lawns sprouting croquet hoops would sit elegantly in front of colonial mansions. Old men would weave silk at the roadside, offering a demonstration in return for a smile. An orange-robed holy man would sit in an impenetrable state of heavy trance. Yoga students would gather on the grass for mugs of *chai* and meaningful conversations concerning *The Bhagavad Gita*. The resident Maharajah would cast a benevolent and watchful eye over all of this from his palace turret.

Well, I did pass a statue of Gandhi. Of his head anyway. I caught a glimpse of it between the arms and heads of three men precariously balanced, along with some brown paper packages, on a bicycle. They were about to be run over by a rickshaw, which in turn was playing a game of cat and mouse with a truck. And there was a strong smell, not fragrant sandalwood but the combined odour of pee, petrol fumes and millions of over-heated bodies. Kiosks, concrete bungalows and cows had replaced the colonial buildings and gently sloping lawns of my imagination. Mysore had all the chaos and pollution of Bangalore but little of the glamour. The advertising hoardings reflected this shift – from whisky to washing powder.

Things looked up when I arrived at the Southern Star Quality Inn – an ode to the seventies – all marble floors, chandeliers and big brown leather sofas. I was thrilled. I would become a white-suited Bianca Jagger, Mick on my arm and the world at my lotus feet.

I took a leather seat in which to watch the hotel's conference room transform into a disco den – at six o'clock in the evening. Lights flashed, beats thumped and disappointingly middle-aged, potbellied men vied with each other for the title of 'Greatest Dancer'. This was not the seventies of Studio 54; there was no Bianca Jagger astride a pure white horse. No Halston or Gucci or Fiorucci. No sexual spaghetti of trans-vestites, transsexuals, gays, straights and bisexuals. Only Crown Paint salesmen from Southern India on their annual conference.

I could see how this was going to go – when the music was turned off several hours later the hotel would become a vicious scene from *Salesmen on the Rampage*. The Crown Paint guys would be drunk, very drunk, and looking for Woman. It was time to go and find myself some yoga students. Caroline had just come back from a month in Mysore and recommended that I go straight to Ortario and Magdali's Café – the handsome Chilean and his French wife were two of Guruji's senior students and the place had become a popular yoga student hangout.

The trip to the café hadn't had the desired effect. Instead of leaving Ortario and Magdali's feeling that I had found my spiritual homeland

I had been very unsettled. I slept badly and woke the next day still uneasy about the conversation with Shanti, Greg and Lisa. It was painfully obvious that I had a lot of work to do on my quest to become a Yoga Goddess – it wasn't going to be easy to put more than a decade of talking marge and drinking Pinot Grigio behind me, and frankly, at this precise moment in time, I was wondering what I had found so wanting in these pursuits – but I was here to find a new life and I needed to put these old ways firmly aside. I was here in Mysore, I was going to meet Mr Venkatesh in one hour's time and I was determined that it was going to be great.

Stepping out of the air-conditioned comforts of the Southern Star Quality Inn into the furnace of an Indian winter, I gave a waiting rickshaw driver the address for Mr V's school, the Atma Vikasa Centre of Yogic Studies. After a geography summit meeting involving half the drivers waiting in line outside the hotel, he agreed to take me, for 300 rupees. Again this seemed excessive, but I decided that if he knew where it was it would be worth it. I didn't want to be late on my first day.

'So hot,' I said, fanning myself as I stepped into the tinsel-lined pink interior.

'Not worry, madam. Air con when move.'

As the hot gritty wind blasted my face, my stomach tied itself in knots – we narrowly avoided two elephants walking the wrong way round the roundabout and more grumpy cows grazing in the middle of the road, their stomachs painfully swollen with plastic and paper. A few barefooted men in tattered *dhotis* walked well-heeled dogs – Poodles, Saint Bernards and Alsatians. Better dressed men busied themselves on street corners doing nothing very much, and the few women out in public walked purposefully in their brightly coloured nylon saris as they balanced entire households on pretty heads decorated with fresh strands of jasmine. They stopped occasionally to buy from forlorn kiosks that sold washing powder sachets and packets of crisps that were past their sell-by date alongside bunches of shrunken, black bananas.

Slowly the sound of radios blasting out high-pitched songs in an indeterminable language and rhythm receded and we found ourselves, I think quite by chance, in Saraswathipuram, the quiet, well-to-do eastern suburb that housed Mr V's school. The lady on reception at the Southern Star Quality Inn had told me it was only about a mile from the hotel but it had taken nearly an hour to get there by rickshaw. I was only just in time. Still it was precisely where Mr V had said it would be – 'exactly opposite the Nalpak restaurant, Kuvempunagar Double Road'.

I waited nervously on the low brick wall outside the unprepossessing school. I had heard that Mr Venkatesh was not only a 'Rubber Yogi' but also something of a perfectionist. Would I live up to his standards? Would he be a complete ogre? I was very relieved when he came to collect me – his manner was gentle and polite, and he looked like a slender Clark Gable, sporting well-oiled black hair, olive skin and a neat moustache.

We sat cross-legged opposite each other on the concrete classroom floor as he explained that I would be starting with the beginners' series and that I could expect lots of individual attention. I had a pretty full daily timetable: *asana* classes at six-forty-five in the morning; ten o'clock *kriyas* (week four onwards); eleven o'clock bodybuilding and massage; and *pranayama* at four-twenty.

A dignified, thorough and kind man, he did what he could to put me at ease, but there was some bad news. I would have to chant at the beginning and end of the class, and at the start of each round of sun salutations. There were twelve rounds. This wouldn't be so bad if I could have chanted with everyone else but the idea was to do it on your own. Two problems:

Firstly, I am tone deaf. At the request of my workmates I had only mimed 'Happy Birthday' to my marge client. I once went to a singing class for the tone deaf but a man from BBC Radio Four turned up challenging us to complete the course by singing live and solo at the Albert Hall. I never went back.

Secondly, the chants were long and in Sanskrit and were displayed on a wall far, far away from my mat. I wouldn't be able to read them. I had decided India would be a good place to give myself a break from contact lenses but Mr V told me that wearing 'opticals' was not a very good plan in class – especially when hanging upside down.

More bad news. I had thought that stepping onto my yoga mat three times a week in London was nothing short of a miracle but I was clearly going to have to step things up if I was to please Mr V.

'I am observing that many yoga aspirants are practising three times a week only. I am observing much lacking of discipline in my students. So I am starting my classes every day. You will be coming on time, ten minutes early is correct. You are waiting for me outside the practice room and I am telling you to come in. If you are late you are missing class. You are coming at six-forty-five every morning except Saturdays.'

'So Saturday will be my day off?'

'No, Saturday you will be starting at six-fifteen as I am finishing with adult aspirants sooner. The little children all are coming after your class; much noise and commotion.'

I would of course try to embrace the dawn but I was concerned that I wouldn't be able to find a rickshaw driver to embrace it with me. The one that had brought me to Saraswathipuram hadn't seemed to like being woken up at nine. I certainly didn't fancy tapping him on the shoulder at six.

He went on to describe the weekly timetable. I panicked at the thought of the *kriyas* – cleansing techniques involving salt water inhaled through my nose and drunk in large quantities to make myself sick. Perhaps there was an alternative plan. Perhaps I could move closer to union with the divine by scrubbing extra hard with soap and hot water on those days, and eating only vegetables?

Mr V concluded: 'Remember, yoga cannot be perfected in an hour, a day, a month or even six weeks. It is taking very many years or life-times. Never trying to take a short cut.'

He suggested finally that I purchase an Atma Vikasa Centre of Yogic Studies T-shirt. Ever eager to please, I did so, even though it cost me ten times the Indian market price – presumably because it offered so much spiritual coverage.

A last piece of advice followed: 'Lucy, when you are upside down you must not be letting the T-shirt to fall over your head. Please be tucking in at all times.'

And then he gave me the rulebook. There were forty-three rules governing the practice of yoga at Atma Vikasa, which included some useful advice:

'Rule 3: When the atmosphere is chilly and cold, when it's foggy and in a field, one should not practise yoga *asana*.'

'Rule 11: During the practice of yoga, one should breathe only through one's nostrils and not through one's mouth. One should not forget that the nose is provided for breathing and the mouth for eating.'

'Rule 34: While studying, there should be a distance of 14 inches between the book and the eyes.'

'Rule 36: To practise concentration of mind abstinence from sex is essential. Reading novels and seeing films that provoke sex impulses have to be avoided.'

There were those who would disagree. I remembered that Richard's *Tantric* friend Osho had said that sexual orgasm can be a meditative experience. I decided to keep an open mind.

There was also unlucky rule 13: 'Eschew smoking and alcohols. These, in addition to harming the mind, may bring in their wake bodily ailments.'

This was going to be a tough one. I am from a home in which five to five in the afternoon is five to gin. As a child it took me a long time to learn that if I was playing at a friend's house, I must ask for Ribena, not red wine.

I wondered for a moment if I should have read the rulebook before I handed over the money. I decided that if I did end up breaking any of the rules I would claim that I never got to read them because a goat ate them.

The next morning I was outside the classroom door at six-thirty waiting for permission to enter. It was dark and cold and I shivered. Bang on six-forty-five, Mr V called me in and motioned to an empty space. The good news was that the senior students had all been going for at least an hour so the room was hot. The bad news – I had an experienced audience. Mr V sat on the end of my mat and sang the first two chants with me. The first chant concerned leaving behind darkness and moving towards the bliss of eternity. The second one offered praise to the sun god:

OM sapthashva rudham Nakshatra Malam
Chaya lolam chandra palam gagana sanchari
OM Bhaskaraya Namaha.

My voice was so tight I thought I might choke, but with Mr V's help I struggled through. He was kind but it was clear that I was most definitely letting the side down. The girls singing their closing chants sounded like fair handmaidens singing odes to bluebells in a meadow bathed with dewy dawn.

Mr V watched me complete seven rounds of sun salutations. It was an unnerving experience – I had never felt so intently watched on my mat before. Unfortunately he found much to correct. 'This is not perfect, do it again' was his usual verdict.

It was funny – the more he told me I was performing the postures imperfectly the more imperfect I became. I got hotter and hotter and more and more anxious. He was occasionally distracted by someone else's imperfect technique but unfortunately he kept coming back to me. I wondered whether I had been doing everything wrong for the past four years or whether Mr V had higher standards or whether the unfamiliar sequencing of postures, strange surroundings and early start were putting me off. Or were my nerves making me stiff and unfocused? Or perhaps all of the above. Mr V asked me to stop when I finished the salutations – normally they are treated as a warm-up to everything else so it felt odd to finish at this point. Half of me was relieved – after all it had taken me an hour to do these seven rounds – and the other half of me was frustrated. I wanted to get going and learn the whole series.

I spent the whole of the first week feeling disappointed at my rate of progress. I had dreamed of showing my fluency in the universal language of yoga – a language that, once mastered, enables you to throw a yoga mat down anywhere in the world and feel at home. Instead I seemed to have regressed to the vocabulary of a two-year-old, as if I was still reading from the handwritten flash cards with which my father taught me to say 'the cat is on the mat'.

I had to learn to live with my frustrations. I spent the whole of the first week trying to perfect these sun salutations. Mr V promised that once he was happy with my progress in this area he would teach me three new *asana* every day. This would continue until I had learned all forty-four in the series, and only then would he give me the coveted illustrated sheet with all the postures.

Bodybuilding classes were also a cause for concern. In my first session Mr V instructed me to stand with my feet apart, placing one foot in front, my knees slightly bent.

'Bend your elbow and make fist with right hand. Placing left hand over right ... No, left over right ... Yes, now you are doing it correctly ... Now, be creating resistance by pushing down on the right hand with the left hand. Trying to raise your right hand ... You are not trying. I can see. This is not perfect. Come on. Really try ... Push. Push. Push! Now do it again, ten times only.'

I had a nightmare that night in which I had to walk down a dark alley to a sweaty room above a furniture store, a long way from the yoga centre in middle-class Saraswathipuram. Two ex-gangsters were living in exile there because a Post Office robbery had gone wrong, leaving a man dead and a price on their heads. Des 'The Matador' Jones would stand over me as I performed a hundred stomach crunches, and Jim Diamond, brought up in a Barnado's orphanage in Whitechapel, would have me lifting dumbbells three times my size.

The other bodybuilding students, all men, were much more advanced. There was a Cat Stevens lookalike from south Carolina. He had kind brown eyes, a wiry beard and wore the white cap of Islam. He worked as a carpenter back home. I didn't know how big his biceps were when he first arrived but he certainly had some good definition now. I could see them rippling as he supported his entire body weight on one hand and then the other, swinging his legs through a full 360-degree circle under whichever hand wasn't on the ground.

Joseph, a softly spoken, dreamy-eyed gap year student from Kentucky, wasn't quite at this stage yet, but he could do the preparatory exercise – supporting himself on his hands, lifting both legs up at a 90-degree angle to the floor and staying there for several minutes, apparently in a blissed-out state of complete relaxation.

Antoine, a short, sharp-nosed, sinewy Parisian, could lift himself from 'firefly pose', or *tittibhasana*, in which the back of his knees rested on his shoulders, up into *adho mukha vrksasana* – handstand. He used to do this five times even though Mr V said that 'only once is necessary'. Sometimes Antoine would throw a *garudasana*, 'eagle pose', into the handstand, tucking his right ankle behind the left. Other days he felt the need to stretch out his legs to 180 degrees while in handstand, or if the studio was crowded, he would show some consideration by squeezing himself into the more compact version – *baddha konasana* in *adho mukha vrksasana* – with his knees out wide, but his feet touching, drawing into his groin. As I watched this performance I wondered if I should introduce him to Shanti. I decided not to bother – they would surely find each other without my help.

Under Mr V's watchful eye I began with some rather more basic exercises. I performed shoulder-building thumb and finger locks. I worked against the wall, pushing hard with my palms as if to knock it down.

'Pushing back with force, Lucy.'

I rotated my arms in circles – clockwise and then anti-clockwise. I stood with my feet apart and rose onto my tiptoes and into a squat.

'Not curling toes into floor for balance. Balance is coming from the navel at all times.'

I attempted to stand on one leg, holding the other one at a 90-degree angle to the floor, clasping the big toe with my middle and index fingers.

'Raising eyebrows not helping raising leg.'

The massage class wasn't quite what I'd had in mind – instead of using long, sweeping strokes and lots of oil to coax each other's bodies into ever more adventurous shapes, Mr V merely instructed us to use the base of the little finger and heel of the thumb to tap tap tap all over our own scalp. Then we tapped one finger at a time. Then we cupped our palms and tapped three times softly, and once more strongly.

The late-afternoons were taken up with the serious business of learning how to breathe. These *pranayama* classes were held in a room tucked away behind the *asana* and bodybuilding room. Like the main part of the school it had a concrete floor, but there were no bars on the windows and the blinds of split bamboo stretched the sun into long shadows across the classroom. The afternoon heat had softened all of us; the rickshaw drivers were fast asleep in their tinsel-lined interiors, the flies had stopped their frantic buzzing, having had their fill of the blackened bananas on sale in the kiosks and even the cows had given up blocking traffic to lie in the scrawny shade of a pollution-choked tree.

We sat in a line waiting. Everyone was there at least ten minutes beforehand; nobody wanted to displeasure Mr V. Cat Stevens took his place at the start of the line-up. He was the most advanced student of breathing as well as of bodybuilding. He sat beside Antoine, whose sinewy chest barrelled out over a powerful set of lungs like a proud pigeon. Then came graceful Mae, an air hostess for Singapore Airlines.

She was clearly a woman used to living in some luxury and only worked first class. She had been in Mysore for two weeks and had already accumulated a driver, a house and a cook. Mellow Joseph sat softly beside her. Then came me.

Mr V explained that *prana* means life force, *yama* means expansion and *ama* means restraint and control. So *pranayama* is the expansion, retention and control of our life force.

'We are working especially on our exhalation,' he said, 'getting rid of twenty per cent remaining in lungs. This is interfering with absorption of energy. You are learning breath retention for maximizing your capacity. Inhalation is coming more naturally.'

I had done some *pranayama* before – mainly on Simon's yoga holidays – but I had never practised it so intensely. In his classes we were usually lying down, and if we were upright it was for short periods of time. Mr V wanted us to sit up straight for twenty minutes and it was causing me all sorts of problems. All those years hunched in front of a computer looking at sales of marge had apparently left me with a spine the consistency of yellow fat on a hot day. I would veer off to the left and then the right. I would tilt forwards and then backwards. I would circle from side to side. All in an increasingly desperate attempt to escape the shooting pains in my back. Poor Mr V was up and down like a yo-yo, realigning me with the gentle pressure of his wooden stick.

At least the first of the breathing techniques didn't appear complicated – just a question of inhaling deeply, pushing out the tummy and then the chest, to get as much air as possible into the lungs. This had to be done smoothly and without pauses. Then I had to exhale until I had got the last twenty per cent of air out. Again no pauses and no jerking movements.

After ten minutes of this I began *anuloma viloma* or 'alternate nostril breathing' in order to balance my sun and moon. The idea was to close one nostril off with the thumb and inhale through the other one. Then to close both nostrils and hold the breath. Then I had to exhale through the opposite nostril to the one I had originally breathed in through. Then inhaling through that same nostril and repeating the whole process twenty-five times. It was easy to get confused. Which nostril was I on? Was I breathing in or out?

The course also involved a thorough immersion in the *bandhas*, which were, Mr V explained, physical locks that help to direct *agni* or 'fire' to any waste matter that may block the flow of *prana*. He placed special emphasis on *uddiyana bandha*, the 'flying up' lock at the abdomen, otherwise known as 'a lion to the elephant of death', such was its power. The *bandhas* would be taught in isolation to begin with, but eventually we would be able to put *uddiyana bandha* together with *pranayama* and the other two major *bandhas* (the chin lock *jalandhara* and the root lock *muladhara*).

Cat Stevens told me of the tradition that says if you open up *jalandhara bandha* in a controlled way you liberate *amrita* – 'the nectar of immortality' – and you live in a state of bliss, healthy and strong, with eight magical powers at your disposal. If you open it without being ready you die in twenty-one days.

It seemed unlikely that I would open it up too fast given my current rate of progress – especially as Cat Stevens said that under normal circumstances it takes twenty years to raise energy from *muladhara bandha* to *uddiyana*, let alone get it up to the chin *jalandhara*.

Of course I got stuck at *uddiyana bandha*, so there was no chance of doing any damage to either *jala* or *mula*. I had to roll up my large T-shirt so Mr V could observe my efforts but there was nothing to see. I was supposed to lift the abdominal muscles upwards and inwards under the diaphragm wall, but they stayed resolutely where they were, not moving an inch, except possibly outwards and downwards. Mr V tried everything; he even had me lie down, thinking it might be easier for me to find my *bandha*, but no. Nothing. Nada.

I put this difficulty down to my family inheritance: 'My mum, granny and I all have the same pot belly.'

But Mr V wasn't having any excuses: 'So, this is your chance to be reversing family genetics.'

I watched enviously as the boys lined up to reveal their perfectly formed *uddiyana bandhas*. Cat Stevens, Antoine and Joseph could even do *nauli*, the advanced version, which stimulates the digestion and keeps the sex organs in full working order. They stood in a row with their feet apart and practised alternate contractions of the muscular columns on either side of their navel. Their muscles churned – moving from left to centre to right in one gorgeous, smooth motion like a rippling wave.

I took to learning my chants poolside, where I could meet other yoga students. The Southern Star Quality Inn's pool was a favourite post-class meeting point. The hotel had introduced a special day rate for yoga students keen to warm their aching muscles on a sunbed amongst the palm trees.

I set to learning the first chant, which I had first performed with Mr V. According to the rulebook, this one would 'take me to *sat* (permanent reality) from *asat* (ephemeral or transient existence), from darkness to light (knowledge of Truth), from (the predicament of) death to immortality'.

OM asatoma sadgamaya
Thamasoma Jyotirgamaya
Mrithyorma Amrithangamaya
OM Shanthih Shanthih Shanthih
Sri Gurave Namah.

'OM' was familiar. We sang it at the end of class in London. Simon had explained: 'OM is the sound of the heart *chakra*. It's the original sound of the universe and reminds us of our place in it, opening us up to the divinity within ourselves.'

How to remember the rest of the words? I decided to use the process I had developed when learning unfamiliar biology terms at school. *'Toma'* was like roamer, *'sad'* was, well sad, and *'gamaya'* rhymed with Yamaha. 'OM asa roamer sad Yamaha,' I hummed.

It was as I was working out what might rhyme with *'thamasoma'* that I met Ben. I had spotted his hard, tanned body glistening with water-resistant oil as he climbed out of the pool, and was delighted when he came and sat down next to me.

We sat in silence for several seconds.

I was busy rehearsing various opening lines when he turned and asked me, with a look of camp insouciance: 'Where do you stand on Christina Aguilera?'

Bollocks. Bloody bollocks. We would just be friends then.

'My name's Ben, by the way. Pleased to meet you.'

'Lucy. Likewise.'

Although I was initially disappointed that we would never be more than mates I was happy to be in Ben's gang, even if he was only doing the occasional yoga class and would be in Mysore for just two more weeks. I loved being bathed in the full and glorious Technicolor that followed him wherever he went.

Deciding that we should broaden our musical horizons beyond Christina, one day we decided to take a trip into town. We found a tiny record shop full of teenage boys. Within minutes Ben had persuaded the seemingly strict and portly proprietor to put on '(Hit Me) Baby One More Time'. The whole shop erupted; twenty teenage boys surrounded Ben as if he were Britney herself. Every single one of them knew every single lyric. Together they became the class of 1999, over-the-knee socks, white shirts knotted high on the chest and hair in bobble-tied bunches. I was dying to join in but there wasn't room. They gyrated and wiggled, sweaty male body to sweaty male body, one seething, unified mass of hormones gone wild, an acid trip of colourful chaos. It was such a relief to see people letting go of their *uddiyana bandhas* – and finding their own unconventional way to that much sought-after state of cosmic bliss.

By the end of our first week together Ben and I were firmly bonded. We even had his and her poolside positions. I took the left, the shade of a palm tree reducing the glare that bounced off the white pages of my chanting sheets, and Ben had the right, a sunny spot from which to observe the pool and its occupants.

One afternoon a shadow, not a palm tree but almost as tall, moved across us. Before Ben could protest at the momentary loss of tanning time, the burning hunk of blue-eyed Norwegian love that I came to know as Erik, had bent down and taken the sunbed next to him.

They had met the day before at V. Sheshadri's yoga school. Sheshadri, gold medal winner of many international, national and state yoga competitions, had a small but loyal following that appreciated his strong adjustments and tendency towards personal demonstrations of hard-to-attain yoga poses.

Erik announced that he had missed that morning's class because he was feeling 'a little full moonish'. 'It's the moon energy, it's mad for me today,' he said. 'It affects my *nadis* and now they're too open, I am too sensitive to others.'

I nodded sagely.

'What's a *nadi*?' asked Ben.

'It's an energy channel,' explained Erik. 'We have seventy-two thousand of them. Our life force circulates through them. And every one of mine is spinning out of control. I feel so uncomfortable, a little faint. I should get out of this heat.' He got up suddenly. 'I will see you guys later. I need to go and lie down. Maybe I will drop by Krishna B's for some healing. By the way I am going to a party tomorrow. Fancy dress. Come with me.'

Erik gave Ben the address and walked slowly away – his pure white linen shirt billowing out behind him, the perfect counterpoint to his faded blue jeans and tousled blond hair.

'I think he likes you,' I ventured, as the last billow of white shirt disappeared around the corner.

'He's only human,' Ben replied.

The party was held at the Post Office House – the coolest of Mysore's yoga houses and so called because it was next door to the real Post Office, a huge operation that seemingly employed half of Mysore.

Although it was a fancy dress party there was no need for the Post Office House to get dressed up – it was already cunningly disguised. From the outside it could be mistaken for a *Miami Vice* drugs den, with hooded windows, a bleached-out balcony and a huge and hungry Alsatian owned by the landlady. Inside, a warren of rooms leading off a dimly lit sitting area had replaced my imagined U-shaped white sofas and mirrors stacked with cocaine. Floor cushions and mattresses warmed the concrete floor for the ten or so yoga students artfully arranged upon them. I waved at Shanti, who was in her favourite position – legs at 180 degrees. She was eating some daal and rice from a banana leaf. She didn't wave back.

All Post Office House tenants are young, talented and beautiful, that much was clear at first sight, but the weird thing about meeting people in fancy dress for the first time is that you don't know how much of their dress is really them and how much of it is fancy. We had met Erik before so we knew that he really was a better-looking version of Justin Timberlake. However, Cat Woman turned out to be a shy but iron-willed Connecticut bookshop assistant called Helen. Mowgli, complete with tiny body, shiny dark hair, loincloth and tan, was a Political Sciences student from Berlin. Ed was a bald-headed giant Pennsylvanian, a benevolent Michael Stipe in a sari. He was studying yoga and ayurvedic medicine. The sari was on loan from the beautiful hostess Heidi. Her hair was so well oiled, and her bindi so perfectly placed, that I initially mistook her for an Indian. However, the guttural German accent was rather at odds with the gliding walk and manners of an Indian princess. Perhaps this was why she didn't say much, concentrating instead on being a domestic goddess and serving up the daal and rice.

Ben dashed my hopes of hearing some traditional sitar music. He had secretly bought with him Britney and Christina's entire back catalogue, and far from causing offence to the hostess, Heidi, Cat Woman and Ed turned out to have a neat line in Britney moves. These were always executed in close proximity. In fact, several hours later the trio were still inseparable and retreated to Heidi's bedroom at regular intervals. Perhaps Cat Woman was helping them with their saris. Certainly they were still having trouble with their final adjustments as they rejoined the party.

Exhausted by my dance-floor efforts at keeping up with Mysore's finest yoga bodies, I retired to the cushions. As I watched Erik and Ben doing a Britney and Justin duet, circa the date they first met when Britney was still a virgin, someone started stroking my hair. It was Bill. I had spotted him earlier in the evening and although I was unsure of his hair, which was long and straw-like, I decided that it was probably, hopefully, part of his pirate fancy dress outfit. He had just returned to the Post Office House from a two-week yoga vacation at the Sivananda Ashram in Kerala (the place where Caroline, my London classmate, had had her spiritual epiphany whilst cleaning the toilet) and was full of tales of the bliss to be found there. Eager to find out more, I suggested that I come by for a mug of steaming *chai* in a couple of days when it was a bit quieter and we could talk properly.

When I returned to the Post Office House the following day (why waste time?) I was relieved to find that Bill had the very short golden locks of a teddy bear. Now that his hair wasn't getting in the way, I could also see that he had come-to-bed, baby-blue eyes and a roll of a walk. He invited me to lie with him in the huge hammock that he had brought back from Kerala. He told me that he had been travelling for seven years on the back of the money that he made as a contract fireman in Colorado. He had gone to the Sivananda Ashram as a rest from the gruelling effort involved in being an *Ashtanga* student.

'Man, it's a beautiful place, it's in the foothills of the Western Ghats and so peaceful – apart from the lions in the park across the lake – they just shag the whole time. Made me feel quite horny just listening to them. We did yoga down by the lake, meditated, swam – avoided the crocs. Cool people, too. Very cool. Very beautiful, especially the Brazilians. Man, they are beautiful.' Bill drifted off to another, more private place.

'Is it run by Brazilians?' I asked, trying to bring him back to earth. 'Isn't that unusual for an ashram?'

Bill laughed. 'Actually it's run by an Italian, a senior disciple of the founder Swami Vishnu-devananda. Vishnu-devananda was a disciple of Swami Sivananda, who had an ashram up in Rishikesh and taught a synthesis of different yoga paths. Swami Sivananda set him a mission back in the fifties – to bring yoga to Westerners – so he went to the States and Canada and came up with the idea of yoga holidays as a way to introduce them to the practice. Actually I found the yoga a bit unchallenging but it didn't matter, it was just a great place to hang out.'

I put it on my list. Next stop, if Richard didn't show up, which, given the rumours about the cocktail waitress, was looking likely.

I asked Bill about life in the Post Office House.

'Oh man, it's so cool. I have lots of sisters back home and it's like being back there. The women here look after my every need. Helen attends to my yoga, Heidi looks after my health – she's an ayurvedic student, you know – and Lisa's an air hostess and organizes my life.'

I could see that there was most definitely a vacant position in amongst these women and wondered why it was unfilled. I decided to apply myself to getting the job. Knowing that there were probably lots of interested girls, I decided to do some queue-jumping and pulled out my secret weapon – my John Denver *Rocky Mountain Collection*. We rigged ourselves up so that we had one earpiece of my Walkman each and snuggled up to listen to John evoking memories of country roads, the sunshine on his shoulders and rocky mountains high. Bill's eyes misted up and he pulled me close. I decided in that moment that I loved country boys. I would follow him back to Colorado. He would build us a house on a ranch, and I would raise horses and strong boys who would tease their old mom as I cooked them their favourite corn fritters with buffalo wing sauce, and blueberry pancakes.

Afterwards he gave me a ride back to the Southern Star Quality Inn on his motorbike. As I wrapped my arms tight around his reassuringly strong chest, I began to worry that if Richard did arrive, it wouldn't be a very appropriate moment.

I needn't have concerned myself. I checked my email the next day:

To: Babe!
From: Richard

Babe! Boiler needs a spare part. Has to be ordered from Germany.
Will be another three weeks. Tops. Promise.
Remember – Shakti rocks!
Boom Shiva!
R x

Hmmm. The only thing was – I really wanted to find somewhere else to live. I had been hoping that Richard would take me to one of the tucked-away yoga student houses he said he knew of but I couldn't wait any longer. Ben was quite happy at the Southern Star Quality Inn, he was only in Mysore for a short while, but I was growing ashamed of my comfort levels. I couldn't stand another day of fluffy towels, hot water and proper toilets. I needed to explore the real India.

Unfortunately there was no room at the Post Office House and I hadn't heard of any vacancies at any of the other yoga student hangouts. That left the Kaveri Lodge. Although I wouldn't want to stay in another hotel indefinitely, it was a little closer to the real India than the Southern Star Quality Inn, and it would be a good stepping-stone. It had a reputation as a place for new-to-town yoga students to hang out before they moved in together. I checked in the next day.

My room reminded me of an NHS Foundation Hospital, but one with no stars. It had the iron-frame beds of a hospital, the walls of a hospital – fading, peeling, industrial green paint on bricks – and it even smelled of a hospital, despite the burning of twenty-four Nag Champa incense sticks. My clothes, washed in a regulation bucket, began to smell, not of my Jo Malone Tangerine and Melon travel wash, but of tin.

I tried to get to know my fellow students but they were always out doing something else – advanced back-bending courses, sunbathing at the Southern Star Quality Inn or having their aching limbs slathered in oil so that they would be able to go the extra inch in the next class. I was disappointed – I'd had visions of hanging out in a big sitting room covered in cushions, smoking spliffs and discussing the day's adventures on our yoga mats, but there was no communal area at the Kaveri Lodge and, when the students weren't out, they were asleep – making up for the five o'clock start and two or three hours of vigorous physical activity that had taken place before the Western world had reached for its first bowl of Crunchy Nut Cornflakes.

I tried to shrug. Surely it didn't really matter; the walls were so thin that I knew everyone, really quite intimately, without actually needing to speak to them. I knew Harjit best of all. He was the Lodge's handy-man and deliverer of lukewarm room service *chai*. He had found an extra special bed right outside my room, on a pile of eight old mattresses. No problem, except that Harjit was a champion snorer. Not only that, but if and when I finally nodded off, I'd be woken at four by the mosque, which thoughtfully provided a municipal alarm clock that woke everyone, except Harjit and the rickshaw drivers, who remained curiously immune.

Mr V noticed me struggling to stay awake in class and suggested I take a look at a room being rented out by Cat Stevens's wealthy landlord. It was in a quiet, leafy side street and I should be able to get a good night's sleep.

Mr and Mrs Sharma conducted my interview, with the four teenage children and several unnamed aunties looking on.

'Where are you coming from, Miss Lucy?'

'Where is your husband, Miss Lucy?'

'Why are you single? You cannot be waiting for ever, Miss Lucy. You should be having many, many children. Maybe it is too late for you now.'

'Not to worry, we find you nice Indian gentleman. Good background. He is liking English girl. We are doing astrology to determine compatibility.'

'What are you thinking is the best biscuit in all England?'

'Would you like a Custard Cream? Aunty is recently returning from trip to Southall. She is bringing back a big red tin. We are enjoying very much. Perhaps your family is sending us more?'

What was it with Indian people and biscuits? I had watched in fascination as the Heathrow check-in staff had exercised a campaign of zero tolerance against Indian families with over-the-limit suitcases. When they began the slow process of deciding what to offload, out came, not Marks & Spencer's underwear, but Peek Freans, Jammy Dodgers and Custard Creams.

I was asked to wait outside while they decided my fate. It clearly helped that my father had trained as an engineer – Mr Sharma's own father had worked on the railways. They said that had swung it for them. They gave me the key and I went down to the bottom of the garden, where I thought I had not understood their directions. I ran back to check but they assured me it was the room on the right, opposite the children's swing and Mrs Sharma's rose garden. In fact, it was the only room on the right. In fact, it comprised just four walls and a door. In fact, it was a coalbunker.

They had taken the coal out but without any windows it was hard to see how the planned white paint could really make much impact. I returned to the family sitting room and said I would think about it; it was certainly very quiet and being so close to Mrs Sharma's roses would be wonderful.

Plan B. I had met Mohan at the Post Office House party. He had won lots of yoga competitions as a child and now, a handsome sixteen-year-old with a penchant for Hawaiian shirts, he was being sponsored by a couple in New York to take lessons with Ben and Erik's teacher, Sheshadri. Mohan worked in a silk shop during the day and, as his very own karma yoga programme, he took time off during the afternoons to help students find a place to live. They expressed their gratitude by spending many rupees on fine fabrics and the shop's in-house tailor.

Mohan roared up to the Kaveri Lodge in a rickshaw alive with pink tinsel and the sound of Elvis. Two of his friends had decided to join him and the three skinny boys crowded together on the seat meant for one.

Mohan invited me to 'step inside the Luurve Mobile'. And off the Rickshaw Four went, to the tune of 'Jailhouse Rock'.

After an afternoon of growing disappointment, we drew up outside a house in the downtown suburb of Lakshmipuram. My heart leapt. From a distance the house looked like a grand and formal old member of the British Raj. Paint peeled slowly away from the walls. The creaking, rusting gates opened onto a once-beautiful and now completely wild garden. The landlady waddled down the path to greet me. We went up to the second floor, past row upon row of padlocked doors. 'To keep the monkeys out,' she explained. Here I was at last; the real India lay before me.

She knocked on the door of number nineteen and said, 'Sean is completing yoga studies. Working too hard always on yoga *asana*, now he must go home to Dublin, Ireland. Poorly sick.'

A small, white blond boy stood before us. His face was as pale as his hair. He used the door for support as he struggled to catch his breath. He had been suffering from a very bad tummy for three months and it seemed to me that he might die here. Brown and green stains oozed from the toilet in the corner of the room. Something was alive in there – Sean needed Lieutenant Ellen Ripley aboard the starship *Nostramo*, not Lucy and a garlanded rickshaw.

That was it.

'To the Southern Star Quality Inn,' I cried as I threw myself head first into the waiting rickshaw.

'Yes, lady,' shouted Mohan, Akshay and Taresh, switching the music to Kool and the Gang's 'Celebration'.

The Rickshaw Four retired to the Southern Star Quality Inn's horse-themed Derby Bar. Ben joined us and we proceeded to get very drunk indeed on Kingfisher beer and Baileys. The drinks went straight to our *nadis*, all 72,000 of them spinning out of control. I am proud to say that I managed to stay upright in the saddle. I was the only one. I attribute this to a strict red wine (not Ribena) upbringing, combined with a bottom that had a higher percentage of fat than all of my fellow drinkers put together.

~ 4 ~

'Possessing only what is necessary'

I settled back into life at the Southern Star Quality Inn. I felt very guilty about the fluffy towels, and uneasy that the real India was passing me by, but my timetable was heavy, I had no desire to live in a coalbunker and I wanted to make the most of my time with Ben. We had a reunion every lunchtime – meeting for post-yoga *Paneer* and Diet Coke served on silver trays by penguin-suited waiters whose shirts provided memories of meals gone by. After lunch we took up our poolside positions. I would practise breathing for my 4.20 p.m. class and Ben would keep lookout for any passing talent. Erik often popped by to see how we were but I noted that he always drew up his sunbed on Ben's side.

Sometimes Madge and Guy pulled up sunbeds next to us. They were just as gorgeously glamorous as their namesakes. Madge was a modern jazz dancer and Guy was a DJ and record producer from Walthamstow. They quickly became our favourite poolside accessories, owning a fine line in sunglasses and allowing us to listen to an endless supply of music on their iPods.

They had come to Mysore for a month so that Madge could work with Guruji and heal an ankle injury that threatened to cut short her dancing career. Guy would rest all day and work on his laptop by night, Fedexing huge files – the sound of sitars colliding with Balearic beats – back to the Camden studio every morning. They had a suite of rooms so as not to disturb each other; Madge had to get up for her 6 a.m. class just as Guy was going to sleep.

We were the Sunbed Five, and I was happy.

And then, quite suddenly, one day I became the Single Sunbed.

Guy and Madge were lured by the old-fashioned charms of the far-away Lalitha Mahal Palace Hotel. A Bollywood starlet in Madge's class had recommended the huge suites with marble terraces, and showers that sprayed you from every direction, and the Wedgwood dining room in which white figurines in empire-line dresses climbed the walls and cherubs chased grapes across the ceiling.

Ben decided to move on, too. He had become close to Erik on a day-trip to Chamundi Hill. They had climbed the thousand steps to the temple together and, like true pilgrims, had their photo taken standing next to the 300-year-old bull known as 'Nandi' as they ate ice cream. Now they wanted to spend some time together 'to see where this might take us' and decided to head down to Kerala. They would travel to Kollam where they would hire a one-bedroom houseboat and some boys to punt them gently up the sleepy palm-fringed backwaters. They would stop off at the Amrithapuri Ashram where they would join the 20,000-strong queues for a session with the Hugging Mother. Ben's friend Janet had been and she said that the Mother's hug had made her rather hot but so happy she had cried for several days. They left the same day as Guy and Madge, and I sat on my bed feeling gloomy. I would have loved to go to Kerala, too, but there wouldn't be enough room on the houseboat and, besides, I was only halfway through my six-week programme with Mr V. I couldn't give up now. There were more than a hundred yoga students outside my door – I would simply have to get out there and make some new friends.

I popped round to see Lisa and Bill at the Post Office House that evening. Bill wasn't there – Lisa told me that she had sent him up to Goa to tie his hammock between a couple of palm trees for a week or two. He was exhausted. Some days, if Guruji thought that he could do some of the second series of postures as well as the first, his practice would last for three hours.

Over a cup of *chai*, on the balcony where Bill and I had listened to John Denver songs together, Lisa told me that Guruji had been a student of the founding father of modern-day yoga, Sri Tirumalai Krishnamarcharya. When Guruji began studying in 1927 at the age of twelve, yoga was considered an unsuitable occupation for a householder, who might, under its influence, lose all interest in the world, abandon their family and disappear off up the mountain. He defied expectations and managed to stay firmly rooted in the real world, marrying, having three children and inspiring complete devotion from students who came from all over the world to learn from him. Despite his advancing years, he still rose early in the morning – reportedly only forty-five minutes after his thirty-something grandson Sharath, who assists him at the school. He makes a cup of coffee, teaches from 5 a.m. to 2 p.m., has a short break and then holds a late-afternoon conference with his students. In the yoga practice room, Lisa informed me, his word was law:

Done your knees some damage? 'Your ego is talking.'

Lacking motivation? 'Everyone can practise – everyone except lazy people.'

Hit a plateau in your yogic growth? 'Practise and all is coming.'

Murdering the form of a posture through insufficient attention? 'Bad lady.' (I knew this one.)

Before Guruji moved his practice room to spacious Gokulam, his students' dedication was tested with long waits on freezing cold steps, as the tiny room could only hold fifteen people at a time. I imagined that these gentle dawn hours would be passed catching up on some reading, peacefully discussing one of Patanajali's 195 yoga *sutras*. Not so. Temperatures in the stairwell ran high by all accounts, and Lisa, whose expression was a permanent one of unmelting butter, told me how she had been the victim of 'Stair Rage' when an American student had mistakenly thought Lisa was queue-jumping.

But this dedication paid off. *Ashtanga* students were always the winners of the unofficial but daily 'Best Body Competition' held pool-side at the Southern Star Quality Inn. Clad in tiny and suspiciously well-cut swimwear, the students weaved their way between the sunbeds. Winning first place in the competition was no mean feat. They were fiercely contested and an extra 0.1 per cent of body fat could lose a student the game. I often saw Shanti claiming first prize; the corkscrew curls and green eyes were supported by an exemplary body, long of muscle and so lean you could see her *uddiyana bandha*. Her preferred reward was a well-oiled shoulder massage from the male winner. Greg, whose lankiness always precluded the possibility of a red rosette on his shorts, would sit looking dejected at the opposite end of the pool.

Poolside was also an ideal place to practise a new yoga pose; it offered a flat surface perfect for balancing on tiptoe in half-bound lotus pose or looking blissful in one-legged king pigeon pose, or, as Shanti would say, *eka pada rajakapotasana*. Plus, an added bonus, there were plenty of fellow students to take a long close look at you, if you found yourself in need of another point of view:

'Can you check my hip alignment?'

'Are you sure I am not clenching my buttocks?'

'My stomach may look flat but is my *uddiyana bandha* really pulled in?'

I was still having trouble with *uddiyana bandha*, amongst other things. Mr V was being patient but I could tell that I was not his star pupil.

'Lucy. Please be paying attention. Even when you are doing it correctly it is not perfect.'

My other classmates steamed ahead of me, proudly displaying their human pretzel gene, as mine remained frustratingly hidden. Three weeks into the course and I was still unable to balance on my right leg whilst clasping my left heel to my forehead, all the time breathing in an expansive and joyous manner, and getting closer to union with divine bliss. My lack of progress meant I wasn't going to be the lucky winner of a well-oiled shoulder massage, at least not in the next couple of weeks.

Worse than this I was having a lot of trouble finding anyone whose life didn't revolve around displaying their pretzel gene and taking part in poolside best body contests. I was beginning to wonder if it might be possible that travel could shrink the mind as much as expand it – far from reducing the size of the ego and merging it with cosmic bliss these body contests seemed to be in danger of creating 'Super Me' egos caught up in the extraordinariness of their physical accomplishments.

What I needed was another party – a release from all this pursuit of bodily perfection, a chance to let my hair down again, and, importantly, to see who would be prepared to let their hair down with me. One small problem. There weren't any parties. The 5 a.m. call of the yoga mat dictated a mug of steaming *chai* and a quick chapter of *The Bhagavad Gita* in bed before lights out at nine o'clock. The party at the Post Office House turned out to have been an exception – held on the eve of a 'moon day', a practice-free day for *Ashtanga* yoga students.

Erik had explained this to me before he left for Kerala: 'We humans are a lot like the sea – we are so very watery that the moon influences us. It's like the tides for us, but our tides are energetic and emotional. On a full moon, when it's in opposition to the sun, we are not grounded. We are headstrong and very emotional. We have to go and lie down, or have a massage. The consequences of practising on such a day can be most severe. On a new moon, when it's in conjunction with the sun, we are also in much danger from physical exertions. We feel more grounded than we do on a full moon but too much so – we are heavy and lethargic, unable to lift our limbs from the ground.'

'So what should we do at this time?' I had asked.

'This is a good time to plant vegetables,' Erik had said solemnly. 'They take root more quickly.'

At least the *Ashtanga* students, with their full and new moons, had two opportunities a month to party, even if they didn't take them. Mr V's students didn't have any moon days at all. Mr V didn't believe in them. The *Nauli* Crew spent the little spare time they had practising their techniques for improving digestion and sexual function, and Mae the air hostess didn't have time for a social life – she was too busy finding a new driver since she had fired the last one for lateness and inappropriate body language.

Perhaps a daytime event away from the rigours of a mat or sunbed would be more conducive to the making of like-minded friends. I had heard that Guruji was going to bless Ortario and Magdali's Café. I decided to go along.

As charismatic as ever, Guruji arrived by limo and took up residence on the big old daybed. He smiled from ear to ear and looked as if he were casting out blessings willy-nilly, but his awe-inspiring presence had reduced everyone to complete silence. No one spoke. Not a great way to make new friends then.

I went to sit outside on the step. The garden was in full winter bloom and noisy with the calls of purple songbirds, but nothing was lifting my spirits. I stared at the now bare garden gate. That goat must have eaten the posters. I thought back to the day I had first arrived, walking up the garden path and opening the door onto what I thought would be yoga heaven. I had such high hopes – of finding my soulmate(s) and a guru who would lead me from darkness to light, and here I was several weeks later still fumbling around in the pitch-black. It was very disappointing.

A shaven-headed man with a large dragon tattoo on his chest came and sat down next to me. I explained my issues as we ate our chocolate muffins, baked in honour of Guruji, for whom they were off limits because he could only eat food prepared by a fellow Brahmin.

Dragon Man asked me if I'd read *The Yoga Sutras of Patanjali*.

'Um, some. Yoga is *"chitta vritti nirodhah"* – I know that one.'

'Well, if you read beyond the second sutra you'll find that Patanjali goes on to talk about the *yamas* – the moral codes that govern how we behave to other people. One of them is *aparigraha* – detachment from desires, possessing only what is necessary. Being happy with what you have, with who you are. He says that attachment creates suffering – and here you are suffering. Let go of the idea of finding your friends and they will come. I promise.'

I thought there was probably a lot of truth in what he said, and there was certainly something quite mesmerizing about his manner. Perhaps it was the dragon tattoo, perhaps it was his turquoise eyes, or even the wisdom of Patanjali. Whatever the cause it seemed right that I should focus on the only thing I could change – my own attitude and expectations. I found myself promising him that I would read the other 193 *sutras* and try to move forward from today – 'possessing only what is necessary'.

Well, maybe I would possess only what is necessary from tomorrow. A chocolate sundae probably wasn't on Patanjali's approved list of possessions but what the heck, I needed a boost. I had seen this dessert, a Southern Star Quality Inn special, bring tears to a grown man's eyes. Ed, the Michael Stipe lookalike from the Post Office House fancy dress party, could eat three in one sitting, but then he was 6ft 6in.

I thought I would have to eat alone but there was the chocolate sundae man himself, with Helen and Heidi. It turned out that this was Helen's final sundae. She was leaving late that night to resume her position at the bookstore in Connecticut.

It was Heidi who suggested it: 'Lucy, why don't you pack your bags and come join us at the Post Office House? You can have Helen's old room.'

Dragon Man was right. Only an hour ago I'd let go of all thoughts of possessing friends and here they were flooding towards me. I was being offered a room in Post Office House. My last fortnight would be spent at the centre of student life, the hippest yoga hangout in town. I had hit the jackpot. And Bill would be my flatmate.

An hour later I was handing over two weeks' rent to the landlady with the Alsatian. I didn't even have to have an interview.

'Friend of Heidi, friend of mine,' she said, her broad smile revealing a life-long love affair with *paan*. The combination of betel nut, spices and limejuice had stained her teeth pantomime black and red.

That night the Post Office House held its second party of the season. We ate sweet *laddu* balls in edible silver foil and Heidi's home-made chapattis. She also concocted some ginger cordial as a special treat; I loved it so much I drank two pints. And then, as if that wasn't enough fun for one day, Bill walked in. He was back from Goa.

He beamed from ear to ear, as did I when he lay down on the cushion next to me and started stroking my hair.

Ed called over to him: 'Hey, man. There are only three explanations for a smile like that. You got laid, you got laid or you got laid. Which was it?'

'I got laid,' said Bill happily.

I was glad that I had my back to him.

'Who was the lucky lady?' asked Ed.

'Miucha, that foxy brunette from Brazil I told you about.'

I looked at my brown hair out of the corner of my eye; the bit that was in Bill's hand.

'She's the one I met in Kerala, at the Sivananda Ashram. Wow, she's hot, man. We rented a little hut on the beach. It was the bossa nova – we were in total harmony. Her legs went on and on and on. Those nights were so hot – boy, did we sweat. The way she moved her hips and arched her spine … man, she was a wild cat.'

'Grrr,' growled Ed, and they collapsed in a hysterical mass of play fighting.

I was in danger of getting crushed beneath them so I retreated to my bedroom and shut the door.

Bollocks. Bloody bollocks. I would have been quite content with one soulmate. How come everyone else seemed to be moving from one to the next with such apparent ease?

The next day I got up bright and early. I was out of the house before Bill, and I was resolute. I would crack Mr V's beginners' series. I would work extra hard for the next two weeks, and then I would leave town, drop down to Kerala. I needed a change of scene anyway. Richard had emailed again to tell me he was still having trouble with his boiler, and there was another email, from one of the Cappuccino Gurus, saying that the rumour was he was getting married to the cocktail waitress in her home town of Skegness. A Christmas wedding? Weren't Richard and I supposed to be on a Christmas mini-break, wearing shell necklaces and bark-fibre headbands? Whatever. Somehow I didn't care any more. Hanging out in a hammock at the Sivananda Ashram would be a great way to start the New Year. And who knew? Perhaps I would meet a Brazilian of my own.

Mr V taught me the last three postures. I managed a headstand for the first time. It was pretty wobbly but I was sure he would help me perfect it. He seemed moderately pleased and, true to his word, gave me the coveted sheets with drawings of all forty-four postures.

I left content and went to the silk shop to tell Mohan the good news, and to get some new outfits made up. My capsule collection of mirrored patchwork skirts and Hindu Goddess tank tops were looking a bit tatty and life at the Sivananda Ashram would definitely call for something slightly more conservative.

By early evening I was lying in a hospital bed wearing nothing but a Porn Star 'Nice Pear' T-shirt and pink pashmina in the style of a dog-walker's *dhoti*.

I had made one near-fatal mistake.

I had assumed that Heidi had used Evian water, or at least boiled and filtered water, in the ginger cordial she had made at the party the previous night. Wrong assumption. Heidi believed so strongly in the ayurvedic principle of being at one with the universe that she drank the tap water and firmly believed that others should not be so namby-pamby as to drink only from plastic bottles with tamper-proof seals.

As I left the silk shop, I noticed that my stomach was growing at an alarming rate. By late afternoon it was doing a very good impression of a watermelon. Leaving Heidi performing some restorative yoga poses to a Dido soundtrack at the Post Office House, I hurled myself at the feet of Dr Kumar in his Saraswathipuram surgery. The world had started to spin.

'I want to go home,' cried Lucy aged six and three-quarters.

'Lucy, you are home. You are with me,' replied Dr Kumar.

I looked up into his kind brown eyes. Angels seemed to be dancing on his shoulders.

He summoned a rickshaw and half an hour later I was in the ayurvedic wing of Mysore's hospital. I worried about this, given that Heidi was an ayurvedic student, but it turned out she had misapplied her enthusiasm. Ayurvedic doctors do believe in a dharmic way of life, living in harmony with the greater universe and healing based on natural laws, but they don't believe in drinking Indian tap water.

Ayurvedic doctors also believe that the body has the power to heal itself. What does this mean to a person with water poisoning? No drugs.

Only pomegranate juice and Dr Kumar's personal copy of *Harry Potter and the Prisoner of Azkaban*.

I slipped into a fever. Still the watermelon grew. Time seemed to stop. At some point in my delirium a doctor from the Western medicine wing came in and, like the devil incarnate, offered me antibiotics and a Jeffrey Archer novel.

'Take these and you will feel better by tomorrow,' he said.

I stuck to Harry and the pomegranates, but only on the grounds that Dr Kumar had angels dancing on his shoulders.

And then the melon's waters broke. I had no control over my movements or my mind, which seemed only to operate when it had to get me to the loo. But then I thought of Sean in the old house in Lakshmipuram and counted my blessings. At least my toilet didn't have brown and green stains and was of Western design. At least I didn't look as if I would need the services of Lieutenant Ellen Ripley on the starship *Nostramo*. At least I was hooked up to a drip – even if it did get in the way of my mobility. And at least I had Rega and Indira, my lovely nurses, who came in from time to time and asked, 'What's happening?'

Generally words were not necessary.

I slipped in and out of consciousness and wondered, in my more dramatic moments, whether I might die alone and intestate – who would get my yoga mats? My Calmia Meditation Mist? My Nuala tank tops? In the days of the East India Company, when the average English emigrant lasted a mere three monsoons in their adopted land before pegging it, the company had very sensibly insisted that the employee write a will before they left.

After three days I regained some interest in the outside world. I was glad I had rented a mobile phone from the manager of the gift shop at the Southern Star Quality Inn, even if it did look like an early prototype. I rang Mr V to explain where I was and then I rang Ben. Perhaps he would come back from Kerala and look after me? Could he bring in meals from home like the Indian people did for their sick relatives?

Unfortunately his relationship with Erik had not lasted. There had been an incident with a boy on the houseboat and they had agreed to part company. Ben was now several hundred miles away, enjoying the turquoise waters of the Andaman Islands with an Australian whose knowledge of Christina Aguilera was impressive. Ben agreed to get a message to Erik, who was apparently on his way back to Mysore.

Erik arrived the next day, wearing his signature white linen shirt open to the nipple line, with a pair of perfectly pale-blue denim cut-offs. All long limbs and goldenness, he stretched himself out on the too-short visitors' bed and announced, as his eyes welled up with emotion, that he was feeling a little 'full moonish' again. He had taken on the pain of the universe, having done too much heart-opening in Kerala.

The sight of Erik's familiar face reduced me to tears. The fun had gone out of being a Post Office House student; I had no desire to return. It had all been quite a strain – my body had entered itself in a time capsule without my permission, travelling back to that first yoga holiday four years earlier when I was stiff as a board. There had been no sense of an imminent merger with cosmic bliss and I was no closer to discovering my purpose in life or finding a man to share it with. I felt very disheartened.

It was definitely time to move on. Being paid good money to debate the meaning of singing sunflowers didn't seem so bad. Should I return to advertising, or at least go home for Christmas? I wanted my mum, I missed my dad and there would be plenty of alcohol at home. Or perhaps I should try a different continent? Byron Bay was supposed to be the yoga capital of Australia, had seven beaches and a huge surfer population. Wouldn't that be much more fun?

Erik wanted to give me a Tarot reading to help me make up my mind. Feeling 'full moonish' casts a very pure and singular light upon the cards apparently. He turned them over. Success, Integration, Playfulness and Rebirth would be mine. All I had to do was pack my bags and get on a train to Kerala as soon as possible.

I also got the Compromise card. Now compromise had never been one of my strong points. I'd always been a bit keen on getting what I wanted – which was why the equilibrium that yoga sometimes gave me was so welcome. Perhaps I had to accept that the path to enlightenment wasn't going to be quite as straightforward as I had thought. Perhaps I would have to change some of my expectations. Perhaps India would throw a few more curve balls my way.

Well, whatever happened next, it hadn't been all bad. I might not have earned an A grade in class but I had lived some of my dreams. I had discussed the teachings of *The Yoga Sutras* of *Patanjali* with a Dragon Man and hung out in a hammock with a fireman from Colorado. I had discovered that a full moon could send 72,000 *nadis* spinning out of control and I knew not to drink from a tap.

And actually it would be better to go to the Sivananda Ashram now – they had a special two-week 'Yoga and Ayurveda Cultural Programme' starting on 21 December that included South Indian classical dance and music, ayurvedic massage and cooking demonstrations. Who wanted to be in Mysore at Christmas anyway? I tried not to think about that other plan I had hatched with Richard – the one involving the Andaman and Nicobar Islands – no, two weeks on an ashram would be so much better for my spiritual development than white sand and turquoise seas.

I returned to class to say goodbye to Mr V. He seemed very understanding about finishing early. The only thing I had really missed were the cleansing techniques, the *kriyas*. He kindly said that there was no need for me to do them as the water Heidi had given me would have done the same job.

I paid my £25 hospital fee, mostly the cost of loo roll and pomegranates, gave Rega my lucky mascot cat, hugged Erik and slipped out of Mysore in a white Ambassador with – who'd have guessed it – something approaching 18 per cent body fat.

~ 5 ~

'Much sex is coming, much money is coming'

Matthew, my driver, was fifty-something and very proud of two things: his shiny white Ambassador and his Christianity. Jesus swung from the rear-view mirror, casting peace and goodwill over his bright-eyed disciple and his brown velvet seats.

Encouraged by the sight of a familiar saint, I accepted Matthew's invitation to sit up front. He asked me my name and looked long and hard at my face, a little too long and hard actually, as we nearly hit a road sign.

'You have very good face. Much is coming, Very happy. Very good. You are giving me hand and I am telling you future.'

We were stuck in Mysore's rush-hour traffic – what else was there to do? I stretched out my palm.

'No. Waiting until clear road. Bangalore road very good. Very fast. I do then.'

Once we were hurtling along at 100 miles an hour Matthew relaxed.

He took my hand and gazed at it. 'Yes, lots of money is coming. Not little money. Lots of money. Money no problem. One year from now, no problem.'

He looked again at my face and pressed his hand into the heel of my thumb. 'Very good man is coming. Very good body. Very good face. Very good heart. You will marry by February year next. Very fast. Very good man.'

I was delighted and wanted to make sure I would definitely be in the right place at the right time. 'Where will I meet him?'

'Not Engleesh man. Not England. No. Hand not saying. But not Engleesh.'

'When will I meet him?'

'Hand not saying. Sex very good. Very good. Please you very much. You enjoy – sixty-four times.'

'Sixty-four times?'

'Sixty-four ways. One day one way. Next day next way. Very good.' He grinned broadly.

OK, let's move on. 'Children?'

'You marry February. Seven months later you are pregnant. Girl is first – very beautiful girl – look like her father. Your father very happy. Then boy. Boy very good. He look like you. Study hard. Very good. Very good sex. Very good.'

'Where will we live?'

'You have car after marry. And big beautiful house. Everybody come. Father. Mother. Brothers. Sisters. Everybody very happy. Very good. Your father very happy. Everybody come. Very good.'

'How about my family – any problems there?'

'Everybody OK. No problem. Very good sex. You good nerves.' He pointed at my groin. 'Very good sex.'

Just as I was about to hurl myself from the moving car, Matthew moved into safer territory. 'Drink plenty water. Plenty, plenty. Lemon and honey – little water – mixing. Then putting on face, neck and chest. Man is looking. Very nice.' He blew out his cheeks. 'Like this three times for total six minutes. Then face coming like apple. Very good.' He was keen to reassure me. 'Very good life. First son is coming, then daughter.'

'I thought you said daughter first?'

'Yes, daughter first. Two son. Two daughter. One son. One daughter. Very good. Good sex. Very good sex.'

We had arrived at Bangalore train station. Thank God.

Matthew summed up the key points for me: 'Very good life. Very good husband. Very good sex. Very good money. Lots of money. Very good tip.'

Suddenly everything fell into place.

Train number 6525, the 21.00 Kanyakumari Express from Bangalore to Trivandrum, sat at the platform for a good hour after it was due to depart. The note on the timetable was proven right – passengers were warned that the published time of departure was the earliest the train would leave.

Leaving Mysore I had felt like a prisoner newly released from jail – seeing the world as if for the first time. Now, as I stood in the train doorway, sounds seemed amplified – the hiss of departing trains, the shouts of the *chai* vendors, the excited screams of children. I took in the broad spectrum of Eastern colours and textures with wide-eyed wonder. How come I hadn't noticed these things before? Living in Mysore had felt very insular, the students were almost entirely Western and there had been little exploration of the world beyond the yoga schools. The small details of Indian daily life that I now saw before me held me transfixed. The platform was crowded with the friends and families of the departing. Young women in parrot-green and flamingo-pink saris tried to control uncontrollable children, older ladies looked stern – adjusting their spectacles and tut-tutting at the lack of discipline, important men charged with important business looked on impatiently. In amongst them mingled beggars, *chai*-sellers, railway staff and porters in grubby red uniforms with brass buttons and epaulettes, who stood watching for signs of weakness amongst the passengers with the heaviest cases and no servants or family. Stray dogs were equally watchful, hoping that a morsel of *samosa* would fall their way from a passing hawker's tray.

I was feeling a little nervous about travelling on my own on a night train. There had been reports in the papers of slashed suitcases, knifepoint robberies and even acid attacks on women. I'd chosen not to travel First Class because I'd heard that it was not uncommon for Western women to be locked in twin-bedded compartments with Indian men. I didn't necessarily see this as much of a problem but apparently unpleasantness had been known to result. I had been advised that 'Second AC' was much safer because the compartments slept four and were curtained, not locked. This was true in theory – there were blue-and-white curtains and four bunks – but it looked as though I was going to be in there on my own.

I busied myself with making up the upper-berth bed – a shiny blue plastic mattress sandwiched between two poles and suspended from the ceiling by strips of canvas. My Southern Railways laundry bag proclaimed: 'This linen was washed in a Power Laundry. If you find any bedroll item Tattered, Torn, Stained or Emitting any Foul Smell, please ask the bedroll attendant to replace the same.' No need – it all looked spotless. I chained my luggage to the hooks fitted under the lower berth and tried to relax.

Eventually the train moved off. Gradually the lights of the city faded and we were in the countryside heading south. I could just about make out the signs for the small stations through the filthy, yellow-coated windows, but eventually the rhythm of the train and my exhaustion (I'd only left hospital two days before) combined to send me into a fitful sleep.

I woke early the next morning to the sounds of a large family climbing noisily aboard. My space was invaded and their victory soon proclaimed. I didn't mind, or at least I didn't mind after I'd had a nice cup of heavily sugared tea brought by the *chai* wallah. The morning passed in a flurry of activity led by the four children who were accompanying their mother to an aunt's birthday party in Kadakavur. Soon I was blowing up balloons, holding the baby, posing for photos with the family and shouting '*shanti*' over the din, much to their amusement.

I was very sorry when they left but I only had to wait another half an hour before the train pulled into Trivandrum. I had made a resolution not to sit up front in Ambassador taxis – at least for a few days – and so I was glad my driver decided to bring his mate along for the ride. We left the crowds of Trivandrum behind and started making our slow way along 30 kilometres of snaking, palm-lined roads towards Neyyar Dam, home of the Sivananda Yoga Vedanta Dhanwantari Ashram.

The humid afternoon heat carried with it the smells of Keralan village life – wood smoke, jasmine, eucalyptus and spices. Women with Mohicans made of 3 metres of brushwood walked purposefully along the side of the road, as moustached, podgy-cheeked hirsute men in billowing black leather jackets and gold-rimmed shades roared by. Gradually the *keet*-thatched huts and kiosks selling fat, red bananas thinned out and were replaced by rolling hills and trees heavy with bright mangoes, papaya and low-slung jackfruits. Occasionally the emerald-green flash of a paddy field cut into the hillside would appear around a bend. The car moved in languid rhythm, responding to the soft curves of the roads, soothing the wobbling pink plastic Ganesh (the elephant-headed remover of obstacles and bringer of good luck) on the dashboard and protecting the two mermaids next to him – caught in a plastic bubble – from a snowstorm soaking. The only thing to disturb the peace was the sound of the driver's horn, which he used every thirty seconds, whether there was anything in his path or not.

We pulled off the main road and started to climb steeply up towards the ashram. A silent glassy lake appeared on the right-hand side and scores of children in the red plumage of the National Cadet Corps paraded past us, pointing excitedly at the Ambassador and yelling, 'Hello, aunty!' at the top of their voices.

And there it was, a sign reading 'Welcome to the Sivananda Ashram'. Another sign requested the driver not to hoot. So hoot he did, three times. We had a brief fight over the price, which, despite being pre-paid and therefore fixed, had gone up 200 rupees: 'Madam, suitcase very big – using much gas.'

I bounded up the steep steps as fast as a person with a big suitcase can, and tried not to cry out at the sight of armed guards at the entrance. This was not going to get in the way of my happiness. I could see lush gardens beyond them, and happy people in bright yellow OM-embla-zoned T-shirts. I followed the T-shirts to their source – a busy office full of reassuringly normal-looking people.

As I sat and waited to check in, I watched a small group signing out to go down to the lake. The security was obviously strict here, but, reas-suringly, there didn't seem to be any problems. A tall Englishman with a chaotic face full of nose, crinkles and twinkly blue eyes – the overall effect of which was very captivating – was doing the organizing.

He asked a man called Jusep whether he had his flute. Jusep nodded happily and gave a small demonstration of what might follow once they were out on the lake. His audience stood mesmerized, but I was not so sure whether this was because of the tight white vest and baggy cotton trousers hanging off his jaw-droppingly perfect, deeply golden frame, or the long black hair, big brown eyes and resemblance to Jesus. Everyone clapped.

The man with the captivating face asked a bouncy-haired girl with wide eyes, a big smile and rosy cheeks whether she had remembered 'the sarnies'.

I leaned forward, surreptitiously trying to see what she had in her palm as she showed the man with the captivating face. It seemed to contain several conical packets of Krishna-endorsed *beedis*, tobacco wrapped in leaves. 'And the thermos,' winked the bouncy-haired girl, quietly showing him the tip of a hip flask hidden in her pocket.

'Good, good. All set then. Now, Cartier,' he continued, addressing a late entrant who had just glided in, wearing a long white kaftan and orange cross-shoulder bag, her long black hair scraped back beneath her YSL sunglasses into a perfect ponytail, 'are you sure you want to come? You know there are crocodiles, don't you?'

'Eeuwww. See you guys later,' said Cartier, turning on her bare, perfectly buffed heels.

'Don't get eaten by the crocodiles,' I said, pointlessly, to the passing man with the captivating face.

'Er, thanks. We'll try not to,' he said, looking faintly bemused. 'Let's go, guys.'

I watched the picnicking party leave, hoping that I would be joining them on their next trip. Meanwhile there were three sets of forms to read and sign. I had to promise to obey the ashram rules: not to leave the premises without a pass; not to go to the local cafés; not to do anything to bring the ashram into disrepute; not to drink; and certainly not to eat garlic.

I imagined there might be some room for manoeuvre given the content of the bouncy-haired girl's pockets, but when I got to my room there were more rules posted outside. The ashram required me to 'Keep silence as much as possible, or talk softly when you must. Swami Vishnu-devananda says, "Silence is the music of your soul"'. I was also asked to keep my 'hair clean and neatly combed, brush teeth and wear fresh clothes daily'. Cartier had definitely read the rulebook.

It was pointed out that the ashram's permanent residents observe celibacy as part of their spiritual practice and guests were asked to do likewise. It went further; there should be no physical contact between the sexes, no 'hand-holding, hugging, kissing or massage in the ashram'. I assumed having a massage was OK if it was ayurvedic and I was paying for it. 'Men and women are not to shower together in the same stall.' It didn't sound as though I would want to linger anyway –

the notice advised me to turn on the shower only long enough to wet my body. Then I should switch it off while I soaped and turn it on again to rinse. And finally, no hairdryers. My glee at finding a plug socket in the room was short-lived.

I sat on my bed, trying to ignore the tin buckets in the bathroom and my one-inch-thick mattress. It was much better to occupy the mind with practical issues like what to wear for my first yoga class – ashram rules and regulations decreed no shorts or sleeveless shirts for women, and intriguingly no 'see-through *dhotis*' for men. I was trying on my pyjama shirt, wondering whether that would provide adequate shoulder coverage over a vest top, or whether I would need to resort to one of Mr V's T-shirts, when my first roommate walked in. My initial reaction was one of relief – she was tiny and therefore couldn't possibly snore. I smiled and introduced myself.

'Hello, dear, I'm Millicent,' she said. Despite her strong handshake she looked tired.

'Long journey?' I asked.

'Oh no, just a couple of hours on the bus from Trivandrum. Quite jolly really. The bus got a puncture so I got out my repair kit and we managed a botch-it job to get us to Neyyar Dam.'

Millicent peered at me over small thick round glasses. She wore a plain blue cotton *salwar kameez* and her thick black hair in a bun. She must have been in her mid-fifties but she had the manner of one who had lived and died in the nineteenth century.

'You sound as though you've been in India a while.'

'Actually, dear, I only got here a couple of months ago. I came to do some birdwatching in the salt marshes of the Rann of Kachchh up in Gujarat and then I went up to the Himalaya. I was visiting a tiny monastery about eight hours' walk from Rishikesh. Bit cold but super people. Very interesting. Would you like a cuppa?'

She was holding a gas stove and some ginger tea.

The tiny rucksack was like a tardis: it contained a tin cup, three

Tiffin pots, a pound of oranges and red bananas bought at the market in Trivandrum that morning, a washing line, clothes pegs, a strip of washing powder sachets, two padlocks, a water purifier, sleeping bag, mosquito net, two *salwar kameez* and the sexiest collection of underwear I have ever seen.

'Did you have to pay to stay in the monastery?' I asked, deciding to save the underwear conversation for later.

'Donation only, my dear. Of course I did some work for them; cleaned out some cowsheds and repaired the fence. Basic work, nothing fancy. How about you, dear? Where have you come from?'

I explained that I had been in Mysore studying yoga but decided to leave out the bit about staying at the Southern Star Quality Inn, substituting it for the Kaveri Lodge and a brief spell in Sean's room in Lakshmipuram.

'Quite right too, dear. When in India and all that. Never pay more than a hundred rupees for a room unless you're getting hot water – and then no more than a hundred and twenty.'

I slowly shuffled my latest credit card bill to the bottom of a pile of papers.

The tea made, Millicent set out on her next mission. Scrunching up her copy of *The Hindu* newspaper and pulling out some vinegar from one of the few previously unmined rucksack pockets, she started to scrub. Within minutes I was also down on my knees, evicting spiders and their cobwebs with a broom made of twigs and string. There was dirt everywhere. How did Cartier manage to stay so clean?

Millicent chatted on. 'You know this bathroom is a big improvement on the bathing arrangements at Swami Vishnu-devananda's first yoga camp in nineteen fifty-nine. It was up in the mountains at St Hippolyte, near Val Morin, Canada. There was no plumbing so they made a hole in a rubbish bin, put it on top of a tree and filled it with water. Did you read about it, dear, in Gopala Krishna's book *The Yogi: Portraits of Vishnu-devananda*?'

I had to admit that I hadn't.

She carried on. 'The fact that Westerners were prepared to do this, to leave all their comforts behind, filled Vishnu-devananda's heart with joy. It looked as if he could fulfil his promise to his guru Swami Sivananda, to bring yoga to the West. Well, if they could put up with that, then who are we to complain? We're living in positive luxury, aren't we, dear?'

'Yes,' I agreed reluctantly. I had, after all, seen worse.

'Well then,' she said, smiling over her glasses, 'let's make Vishnu-devananda's heart sing again.'

As we scrubbed our way through the afternoon, I found out that she had travelled all over India with two young children and, after her husband had left her in Kathmandu in the late seventies, raising them single-handedly.

'Stick with me, my dear,' she said. 'I'll show you the ropes.'

The call to dinner was a gong. Millicent and I had worked up quite an appetite with all our scrubbing so we wasted no time in joining the long lines of chanting ashramites sitting on the floor in the overwhelmingly blue Dhanwantari Hall. At the end of the chant we joined in the chorus of '*Jai*', which, Millicent explained, was the equivalent of 'Praise be'. The chant seemed to involve praises to one *Hare* OM, which I took to be the name of the cook, until Millicent told me, with a look of some severity, that it was one of God's names.

The food was brought out in big tin buckets. Rice, poppadoms, chickpea curry and fresh beans were soon piled high on my segmented tin *Thali* tray, and I began the slow process of learning to eat with my fingers. I spilt many chickpeas on my white trousers but I noticed, with some satisfaction, that the orange-clad men at the end of the line, the only people adhering to the 'OM Silence Please' rule, were as messy as me – though the colour of their robes did provide them with useful camouflage.

Millicent tried to reassure me. 'Take heart, dear – when a disciple tried to wipe away the tomatoes which had dripped out of Vishnu-devananda's sandwich, all down his orange sweater, he just smiled and said, "See, even the tomatoes are attracted to me. They want to be with me." Isn't that funny? He was a very funny man.'

I agreed, and hoped it bode well for my spiritual development that chickpeas wanted to be with me, seemingly for ever.

The food that I did manage to get in my mouth was actually pretty bland – probably in accordance with 'Proper Diet' – one of the five principles of yoga outlined in *The Sivananda Training Manual*, a slim booklet I had bought in the well-stocked ashram shop that afternoon. Just as a car needs 'a lubricating system, a battery, a cooling system, the correct fuel and a responsible driver', the body also needs 'Proper Exercise', 'Proper Breathing', 'Proper Relaxation', 'Proper Diet' and 'Positive Thinking and Meditation'.

There was no sign of the picnickers at dinner, but I was glad to see that most people seemed, like them, to be pretty relaxed – very few of my two hundred or so fellow diners were in full lotus position, and there was quite a range of personal styles. A pale, tattooed traveller girl in a nylon dress, pedal-pushers and scooped-up blonde dreadlocks chatted quietly with a burly Australian man in a boomerang-and-koala shirt. A Divine Child with golden hair and One World tank top hid behind the blue pillars, trying to avoid her mother and the chickpeas. A large Indian man, whom I would later know as Ravi, shook uncontrollably at his friend's joke, and Cartier sipped her coconut milk without spilling a drop on her still-spotless white kaftan.

Instead of relaxing in front of the telly for the evening, the ashram's next move was upstairs to the 'Swami Vishnu Devananda Samadhi Memorial *Satsang* Hall', otherwise known as the Shiva Hall. This was decorated with tinsel chandeliers and a giant golden OM – as gaudy as the ads for washing powder in Mysore. Would it wash my spiritual life whiter? Perhaps I'd come up a bright shade of orange?

We sat at the front, beneath a stage emblazoned with Swami Sivananda's exhortation to 'Serve, Love, Give, Purify, Meditate, Realize'. On either side of the giant OM were orange-garlanded pictures of Swami Sivananda and Swami Vishnu-devananda, an earthy, open-faced man who looked as if he were about to burst out laughing. There was also a photograph of him beside his brightly coloured twin-engine peace plane, painted by cosmic sixties artist Peter Max. Millicent informed me later that, according to Gopala Krishna, he was known as 'The Flying Swami' for his peace missions over troubled territories, 'bombing' East and West Germany and Arab–Israeli lines with flowers and peace leaflets. He travelled with a 'Planet Earth Passport' that gave his weight as 'immeasurable', his eyes as 'intuitive' and his residency as 'earth'. I hoped his disciples had the same sense of humour.

I found it hard to concentrate in *satsang*. I asked Millicent what the word meant and she explained that it came from Sanskrit – 'a *sanga* is a company or brotherhood and *sat* means truth or godliness. My dear, we are a company of truth-seekers.' The truth was I was tired. After an hour of meditation and chanting – led by a pale, thin, stooping American *swami* on a harmonium – I was ready for bed. I stuck around long enough to enjoy the chanting of the sweet, soft *Arati* Prayer, 'Prayer of Light', followed by the waving of the *Arati* lamp in front of the altar to denote that the Lord is the light in the sun, moon and fire. The lamp then left the stage, held high by a grey-haired woman in a white dress, and the ashramites took turns to warm their hands over the flame, moving their hands over their hearts and up over the top of their heads.

We walked back to our room. Millicent, having explained that this latter gesture symbolized the purification of the self and the burning of the ego, retired to bed in full black sexpot underwear and proceeded to snore like a trooper.

I finally got to sleep at five in the morning only to be woken again at five-thirty by a gong and wailing temple music from the nearby village, which sounded like Minnie Mouse dancing on red-hot coals. Millicent was already up, making ginger tea.

The day peaked early with a *puja* – a worship ceremony – at six o'clock. It was dark when I walked into the Dhanwantari Hall and all I could make out were Toblerone-shaped rows of white shawls. I took my place amongst them and learned that this *puja* was in honour of Ganesh. Worshipping him would remove any obstacles that might come our way over the next couple of weeks. The ceremony turned out to require our full participation. I was terrified of getting it wrong so I aligned myself with a smiling, jasmine-scented Indian girl, who had been serving chickpea curry the night before. We knelt together in front of an Indian orange-clad *swami* and prostrated, grabbing a handful of what looked like popcorn from a large pile in front of us, holding it to our hearts for a moment then throwing it into the fire. It can't have been popcorn because it didn't pop. No matter. We prostrated again and returned, safely, to prayer position.

It was a different story when we went to be blessed by a whole row of *swamis* and *sadhus* – the men who wander all over India with just a begging bowl and the clothes on their back. These renunciates, living the age-old ideals of the eremitical life, often check in to an ashram for a few days of R&R. There were three of them at the Sivananda Ashram – they had been invited to stay for Christmas, obviously at no charge.

I held out both my hands for the water blessing.

'Right hand only – *at all times,*' came the sharp retort from the *sadhu* with three horizontal lines of sandalwood paste on his forehead. Millicent told me later that the left hand is reserved for the toilet: 'It's a necessary distinction when both eating and wiping are done with the hands. Take care to observe the custom, dear. When in India and all that.'

She also explained that the horizontal lines meant he was a *Saivite,* a follower of Shiva – the lines symbolising God's threefold nature as creator, preserver and destroyer of the universe. That the *Vaisnavites*, followers of *Vishnu*, wear vertical lines of sandalwood on their forehead as a symbol of his preservation and protection, and that followers of the Vadagalai School of Ramanujacarya wear a white U-shaped mark with a central red line. The U is the right foot of *Vishnu* and the central mark is a symbol of his consort *Lakshmi*.

The best bit of the *puja* was coming face to face with the acting *swami*-in-chief – known from that moment on as the Swoony Swami. He was at the end of the blessings line-up and he gave me my first *kumkum*, invoking the supreme power of Devi, the universal mother. I was so taken with his racing driver good looks – a strong, lean body, short dark hair, piercing blue eyes and long, noble nose – that I didn't wash off the red mark he pressed into my forehead for two days. According to Millicent, he had only been initiated as a *swami* recently. Swami Mahadevananda, the Italian head of the ashram and Vishnu-devananda's most senior disciple, was currently in Canada but had performed the low-key ceremony which entailed a life of celibacy before he left, just six weeks ago. I was six weeks too late. Bollocks. Bloody bollocks.

Unfortunately, the Swoony Swami was only teaching yoga to the more advanced students, and those who had been staying at the ashram for a while. As a newcomer I had to join the beginners' class for a few days even though I knew the Sivananda series, having attended introductory classes at their centre in London – an oasis of incense, orange robes and multi-coloured wall paintings of Hindu deities amid the middle-class Victoriana of Putney. I was disappointed not to be spending more time with the Swoony Swami, but the beginners' class had its compensations as it meant walking past the guards and crossing the road to practise on a yoga platform in an idyllic spot by the glassy lake. Even at this early stage, leaving the ashram felt quite an adventure.

John, our laconic teacher, offered instructions, occasionally interrupted by the sound of what could only be the shagging lions that Bill had told me about, who were indulging themselves in the safari park across the still water. John ran his fingers through his hair and took us through the twelve basic *asana* of the Sivananda series. Despite spending a lot of time in *savasana*, the 'corpse pose', the combination of lions, heat and 'pumping deep bellows' breathing of *kapalabhati*, 'shining skull breath', left me feeling pretty spaced out. I wasn't the only one. One girl fainted. Fortunately Millicent, with her first aid skills and smelling salts, was able to put her back together.

Dan, whose blond highlights I had spotted at the *puja*, walked with me across the road, back to the ashram. He proclaimed himself knackered. 'I was kept awake all last night by the bloody orange men. They must have gone to the toilet five times each, hoiking up God knows what, then they were smoking *beedis* and God knows what out the back of the dorm. And Christmas Eve we're going to be up until after midnight with God knows what *puja*. Shouldn't we be asking for a lie-in on Christmas Day?'

'Preferably with an orange juice and a croissant,' I suggested.

'Some sex would make it just perfect,' he replied.

After a late breakfast of *iddlies* – spongy rice cakes – and vegetable curry, it was time for some hard work: *karma* yoga, the yoga of selfless action. Millicent told me that Swami Sivananda had used this yoga to help his disciples grow spiritually by setting Vishnu-devanada to wash clothes in the river, a job far below his caste. Caroline, my friend from London, had her spiritual epiphany cleaning the toilets here. I would surrender to whatever John, doubling up now as 'Head of Karma', asked of me.

He set me to cleaning the vast Shiva Hall floor with the bouncy-haired girl, who turned out to be called Astrid, Jusep and a couple of twigs that had enjoyed a previous life as a broom. To brighten up the task we set to singing. Quickly tiring of 'Like a Virgin', we moved on to the *Live in Satsang* chant book and sang for the first time what was to become our ashram anthem – the very upbeat '*Jaya Ganesha*':

Jaya Ganesha, Jaya Ganesha, Jaya Ganesha Pahimaam
Sri Ganesha, Sri Ganesha, Sri Ganesha Rakshamaam.

We could only remember these first two lines so we set them on a repeat loop, as Astrid performed an accompanying elephant-like movement with her hand swinging down between her legs. At some point '*Jaya Ganesha*' became 'Free Ganesha'. We used the chant as a sort of metronome to keep the beating of our broom twigs steady. I think John was a little surprised at our speed but agreed that we might want to use the routine at the ashram talent show on Christmas Day.

Hard work over, we went to sit in the garden underneath the Cannon Ball, Fig and Neem trees. The long fronds of Travellers Palm waved in our faces, creating a welcome shade. John took up what was clearly his favourite pose – lying propped up on one elbow, between two Ashram Babes. Today it was the turn of the Israeli girls – Ronit and Ronit – slender eighteen-year-olds in cotton trousers rolled low over their hips, tight tank tops and tiny cardies, the height of ashram chic.

To be an Ashram Babe you had to be naturally pretty. Few of the girls appeared to be wearing any make-up and the draconian rules about electricity usage precluded hairdryers, so natural corkscrew curls were the best hairstyle, or else long, flowing, straight tresses that could be swept into a chic ponytail or pinned up into a 'I never bother with my hair' look. I sat silently mourning the day I had let my hairdresser give me a flicky, high-maintenance London cut. I had tried using the hairdryer that morning, covering up the noise by singing loudly, but a power cut – the hand of God? – had stopped me. I was now reduced to wearing my hair in bunches. I thought I had got round the unofficial no make-up rule by using soft 'barely there' colours but Millicent had still called me 'The Make-up Queen' as we had left the room this morning.

The conversation turned to ashram rules. I asked Astrid whether passes were freely available.

'No, they only give them out on Sundays,' she said. 'Otherwise you must take your mat and pretend that you are doing yoga by the lake – you can be gone two hours without anyone noticing. It's long enough to get down to the café by the dam and have a Coke.'

'And a *beedi*?' I asked.

'Definitely you have time for a *beedi*, maybe even ice cream.' She smiled.

I smiled back.

The long, dark shadow of Millicent appeared across the lawn. 'Hello, Make-up Queen.'

My cover was blown. 'Hello, Millicent,' I grimaced.

Astrid, not knowing my roommate very well, told her the subject of our discussion.

'Well, girls. I expect I should disapprove, I really should. But you're in good company. It says in his biography that when Vishnu-devananda was at the Val Morin ashram he had meetings with his secretaries in the local town diner. He'd sit in his shorts and a T-shirt and order French fries and sugar pie with ice cream, which he would offer to share with any refugee ashramites. He was a jolly old sort.'

'Cool,' said Jusep, being a man of few English words.

I wondered if there was any chance the Swoony Swami might follow in his guru's footsteps.

I turned to Cartier, who was sitting underneath a large frond on the edge of the group, engrossed in a magazine. She looked spotless in white linen trousers and her big black YSL shades.

'What are you reading?' I asked.

'Well, it sure isn't *Yoga Journal*.' She turned the magazine over secretively – it was the latest issue of American *Vogue*. There was a rule about suitable reading matter: spiritual books only, no novels. *Vogue* was most definitely a felony.

Charlie, the man with the captivating face, appeared and had soon coerced the Ronits and Astrid into his latest plan – one that involved a place called the Health Hut. They left, leaving John without any babe action. He began to move towards Cartier but something in her look made him abort his mission. After a minute he got up and walked away.

Naughtily I relayed to Cartier the conversation I had with him earlier that day – when he had explained that he spent his winters teaching yoga at Sivananda centres because he found it easier to lead a spiritual life away from home. I had asked him whether he had ever considered becoming a full-time man in orange. He told me: 'I think about sex all the time. A crocodile would have to bite my balls off before I'd become a *swami*.'

I should have slept well that night. I was exhausted after the second *asana* class of the day, which had resembled a *Bikram* yoga session as the temperature soared to more than 30°C, leaving me looking like a sweaty beetroot. I saw Cartier after her advanced class – still perfectly turned out, not a hair out of place – her long, black ponytail swinging over a not too loose, not too tight cream Juicy Couture tracksuit, her leather yoga bag a perfectly contrasting honeyed brown – the undisputed queen of ashram chic.

I had spent the evening in a trance in the Shiva Hall, which had looked magical as candles cast shadows of deities and Dr Ananada Padmanabhan over the golden OM. The Doctor was a master *veena* player who sounded like Ry Cooder, or perhaps Ry Cooder sounded like him – a sort of *Paris Texas* in Neyyar Dam, Kerala. The only thing that prevented me from becoming lost in the lunar landscape of the Mexican desert with Travis, sweating in a cheap, dusty suit and sandals held together with bandages, was the excruciating pain in my knees and hips, born of too much time spent sitting cross-legged on the floor.

Despite the heat exhaustion and the *veena* lullabies, I'd spent another night tossing and turning. The fan was on full blast but its insistent hum, combined with the pain in my hips and knees, and Millicent's snores, left me awake and bad-tempered at 5 a.m.

Still, at least everyone was in a bad mood at breakfast time. There was rebellion in the ranks. Dan hadn't slept either – courtesy of the abluting swamis – and Charlie was pissed off with Dan for washing his balls in the bathroom sink. The breakfast *iddlies* looked delicious and tasted of nothing. Astrid was craving fresh vegetables. Cartier had got her clothes back from the ashram laundry and had found a mark. Only Jusep remained cheerful, leaving the hall to go and play his flute under a Travellers Palm frond.

'I vote we strike for better conditions,' said Dan, militantly.

We all agreed, except Charlie, who looked ready to murder him.

Things didn't get any better for a while. John assigned me to cleaning the girls' dorm toilets and bathrooms. Perhaps he thought that we'd had too much fun yesterday – although I noticed that Jusep and Astrid were reassigned to the Shiva Hall and allowed to carry on rehearsing their broom routine. No matter. I applied myself to the task at hand. I found a mop with more than three pieces of tattered string attached to it, and worked very hard. I really did. I tried singing 'Free Ganesha' to myself, but it wasn't the same without the other two and there was not even the faintest glimmer of a spiritual epiphany, just a lot of hair in the plughole.

I had also worked hard in the 6 a.m. *satsang* but my meditation was marred by an inability to switch off those all-too-familiar mental whirlings, the *chitta vritti*. The meditation instructions painted on the front of the stage, underneath the exhortation to 'Serve, Love, Give, Purify, Meditate, Realize', were very precise and, wanting to maximize my chances of reaching *samadhi* and attaining 'eternal bliss', I followed them to the letter. But no amount of observing the mind as a silent witness, selecting a focal point, visualizing an uplifting object and repeating the *mantra* OM were taking me where I wanted to go.

'Eternal bliss' were definitely not the words I would use to describe the experience. 'Eternal torture' would have been more fitting – caged in with all my thoughts, unable to escape. Why wasn't I making any progress in this area? Why was it so hard to switch off from the constant chatter? OK, so I wasn't thinking about asking the boss for a raise any more or whether anyone would want to go for a glass of wine after class, but this was only because money and wine were not part of ashram life. Fresh mental clutter had simply taken the place of these thoughts – how to move up to the Swoony Swami's advanced yoga class, and how to become the epitome of ashram chic using the current contents of my suitcase (I'd slightly overdone it on the conservative clothing brief to the silk shop in Mysore and the ashram shop didn't have any solutions – the T-shirts were all a little on the large side, the trousers a little too baggy). I would have loved to take a break from these thorny issues but the more I tried not to think the more thoughts came flooding in.

Luckily help was at hand. The Swoony Swami gave a lecture that afternoon on meditation. He told us that 'Freedom is actually the ability *not* to do what the mind wants to do. Of course, it's usually defined as being able to do what you want to do when you want to do it.'

Everybody laughed. We were captivated.

'"Bliss is your birthright,"' he said, quoting Swami Sivananda. Assuring each of us that we 'were put on earth to be happy and fulfil yourself, not to suffer', he urged us to 'commit to finding happiness within yourself. Meditation is one of the most powerful ways of accessing this happiness within ourselves – not just when you are having an ice cream in a beautiful place.'

As per the instructions on the front of the stage, the Swoony Swami suggested that we try practising *japa*: 'focusing on and repeating a *mantra* – a mystical energy in a sound structure'. He went on. 'A *mantra* has a specific purifying, calming and elevating effect – think of it as the tuning knob on your mind, the radio. Which *mantra* you choose doesn't matter, just select the one that connects with you. But,' he warned, 'use only *sattvic mantras* for spiritual development, for example, "*OM Namo Narayanaya*", which is the chant for world peace.'

I adopted *OM Namo Narayanaya* as my own and gave it a go in the evening *satsang*. It started off well – performing a mental roadblock on other thoughts for several seconds. But then it started running away with me, getting faster and faster, eventually taking on the pitch of temple music. Surely a shrieking Minnie Mouse dancing on hot coals was not creating the desired purifying effect? I tried to imagine that I was listening to the Swoony Swami's gentle lilt but Minnie, by now a hyperventilating harridan with charcoal for feet, kept bouncing back into earshot. Perhaps this wasn't the technique for me.

Dr Janarthanan's post-*satsang sitar* performance presented my increasingly stiff knees and hips with another challenge. I really did want to contain my spiritual energy by sitting cross-legged as the Swoony Swami had instructed, but I ended up having to uncross my legs and let it seep out across the floor. Eventually my whole body wanted to seep away, so I moved out of the hall to the corridor that ran alongside, intending to put my feet up on one of the pillars. There was quite a crowd out there – it was hard to find a spare one. Charlie was fast asleep, lying between one of the Ronits and Astrid. Cartier was reading *Vogue* again, and looked as if she should have been smoking a cigarette. I peeked back inside the hall. Millicent was one of the few remaining devotees, her straight back allowing the free flow of spiritual energy up to her bun.

The next day was Christmas Eve. I can claim that it began gently enough, if I ignore the murderous thoughts pertaining to Millicent's snoring that buzzed around my head on the 6 a.m. silent walk to the glassy lake. The National Cadet Corps were out in force, their red plumes bouncing up and down as they ran alongside us giggling and shouting, 'Hello, aunty!' Meeting only our vow of silence, they gave up and goaded each other into ever more vigorous press-ups on stone benches. We sat on the banks of the lake, our backs to the press-up action, and chanted the *Arati* Prayer, as the locals washed themselves and their cows in the rising mist.

We came back to yoga, breakfast and my selfless act of the day –
more toilet cleaning. Afterwards, in need of a bit of 'me' time, I sloped
off to the Health Hut, tucked away at the top of the ashram. Sitting at an
orange wooden bench, I ate a fruit salad, served by none other than
Cartier, who was engaged in her half-hour of selfless action. I contemplated the distant views out towards the foothills of the Western Ghats
and, slightly closer to home, the smoking *sadhus* on the platform at the
back of the boys' dorm.

I was definitely ready for a slow day. The ashram timetable left very
little time for chilling out so I decided to skive off the lecture and afternoon *asana* practice – perhaps I'd go back to the room and have a sleep
while Millicent was having one of her increasingly regular chats with the
Swoony Swami.

Suddenly I was surrounded. Charlie on my right. Astrid on my left.
Cartier watched from the safe vantage point of the juicer.

'All right, doll?' said Charlie, his blue eyes twinkling.

'All right,' I replied nervously. There was something about …

'Got a project for you,' said Charlie.

'I was just going to have a relaxing—'

'I want you to write the ashram nativity play – we'll put it on as part
of the talent show tomorrow night. I'm directing, Astrid is assisting me
and Jusep is playing Joseph. Still gotta find a Mary. OK with you?'

'Well, actually—'

'Great, cheers, see you later. Are you going to the talk on *Kathakali*
this afternoon?'

'No. I was going to have a lie-down. I'm feeling a bit—'

'Good, then we can run through your initial ideas at two this afternoon. Don't worry – just top-of-your-head stuff. Cheers, Luce. See ya.'

I looked out towards the distant mountains and found myself wishing that I were on top of one of them, preferably in a cave wearing
orange and having undertaken a fifteen-year vow of silence.

Dan happened to call in at the hut for a ginger, lemon and honey tea so I co-opted him and Cartier, who had finished selflessly serving, to help me.

An hour later we had produced an expansive eight-scene play, which took in Wembley stadium, Malaga airport duty free, a *dhoti* manufacturing plant in Mumbai, a mountain cave, a girls' dorm, a Fifth Avenue beauty parlour, a New York club and a stable.

Charlie blamed recent budgetary cutbacks as the reason for canning four out of the eight scenes and as many locations. I was relieved the basic storyline remained intact. We had laboured long and hard.

Scene one: Joseph spots Mary in a Fifth Avenue beauty parlour and falls for her instantly. Mary is otherwise occupied discussing ashram chic with her gal pals – orange is the new black this season – and which *swami* should be December's pin-up of the month. But when Joseph bursts through the door declaring undying love, she is captivated and the happy couple ride off on a broom containing several twigs.

Scene two: Mary and Joseph are now a couple and are shopping in duty free at Malaga airport. The relationship is already beginning to fall apart as Joseph's need for *beedis* and Kingfisher beer becomes harder to hide – as does Mary's bump.

Scene three: Beneath a 'Deluxe Ashram' sign sits a Door Bitch – probably a Cartier cameo – whose strict guest list and 'no Birkenstocks' policy keeps Mary and Joseph firmly on the outside.

The couple move onto the 'Very Proper Ashram' sign, underneath which a guard insists that the couple chant either '*Jaya Ganesha*' or the *Arati* Prayer if they are to be allowed entry. Of course, Joseph's drinking problem gets in the way of his memory and they are refused.

The exhausted couple arrive at the Sivananda Ashram and are met by the Swoony Swami, who welcomes them with open arms, so long as they promise to obey all of the ashram rules. He has just got to the bit about *karma* yoga when Mary goes into labour. The labour is long and hard and involves much screaming and blood. She is helped by *kapal-abhati* breathing, but not by Joseph who is being a pain in the butt, so she asks him to leave. The baby pops out and is cradled in a hip-opening yoga pose. Joseph is forgiven.

Scene four: The three wise men, guided by the star of Bethlehem, kneel down beside Mary and utter their wise words – the words the universe has been waiting to hear – their gift for the baby Jesus.

'One thing, Charlie,' I warned, 'at this point we don't know what these words are. But don't worry, we're working on it.'

'That's all right, love, but the ending is weak. You need something with a bit of punch, some balls, audience participation – ideally some kind of singalong.'

Somehow I agreed to have the finished script ready for midday the following day, Christmas Day.

Satisfied with the overall direction of the scenes, Charlie turned his attention to casting. His years of experience in telly meant that he was best placed to decide who would play whom.

Jusep was a natural for Joseph. No arguments there. Then there was Mary. This caused more dissent. I had always harboured a desire to play the most famous virgin in the world. Astrid and Cartier were supportive, but I didn't seem to cross Charlie's mind. His first choice was one of the Ronits but she was uncomfortable with the storyline. Perhaps I would be second choice? Nope. Charlie then suggested Mitzy, a striking Thai beautician living in Stockholm whose tanned skin and chiselled bone structure was a perfect complement to Joseph's. Even I had to admit, when I had finished regressing to the age of seven, that Charlie was right – they looked the perfect couple. Ravi, with his amply proportioned lungs, was brought in to play the baby Jesus. He wouldn't have to be on stage (lucky, since all of him was amply proportioned), as his first cries on earth would be heard from behind the wings.

Charlie gave Cartier and me the task of being Mary's gal pals – I would play the hairdresser as I had a hairdryer and Cartier would sit around painting her nails. Cartier was also confirmed as the 'Deluxe Ashram' door bitch. Charlie decreed that Millicent should be the 'Very

Proper Ashram' guard – a role everyone agreed she had been born to play – and that she could double as the midwife, since she was a first aider in real life. Dan appointed himself narrator. It was hard for Charlie to argue about this, because at least a third of the play was Dan's vision, but I could tell that he wanted to.

Charlie had already worked out that the three *sadhus* should play the three wise men and went off to talk to them about their roles. I retired to the Health Hut to write the full script, and Dan went to his room to choose his outfit – he was favouring sunglasses, gold lamé shorts and a white singlet. Millicent went off to make all the props, reminding me to bring my hairdryer and make-up for the beauty parlour scene ('It's a good thing you're a Make-up Queen, isn't it, dear?'). Mary and Joseph went to have a massage so they would be relaxed for their big roles the next day.

I saw Charlie later on in the afternoon, crouched before the Divine Child's miniature barn, all lit up with fairy lights, giving the three *sadhus* a mini-tutorial on the traditions of the Christian Christmas. The three wise men had gathered round the barn and nodded in fascination as Charlie used pidgin English and the contents of the barn – three model Marys, two Josephs, four baby Jesuses and assorted farmhouse animals plus a monkey – to give them a fully enacted nativity story.

Christmas Eve evening kicked off with a bang. The visiting *Kathakali* dancers, one of Kerala's major tourist attractions, put in an appearance so bling they would have made a drag queen look underdressed. The crowd grew dizzy with the sight of grown men in lurid green and red make-up, the contours of their cheeks extended with moulded lime, white kitchen-cabinet knobs on the end of their noses, wobbling about in hooped petticoats and three-tiered, rainbow-coloured head-dresses. None of us knew quite what was going on but there appeared to be a lot of emotion in the air: the dancers' eyes ran the full gamut, from anger to love and fear, and back to anger again.

By the time they left the stage reluctantly, two hours later, the audience was completely intoxicated. We threw ourselves into a round of carols so energetically that even the thin-lipped American *swami* accompanying us on his harmonium had to smile. We blitzed our way through all the old classics – 'Hark the Herald Angels Sing', 'O Little Town of Bethlehem', 'O Come All Ye Faithful' and even, in a small departure from the usual church service, 'I'm Dreaming of a White Christmas'.

We hit our peak with 'Jingle Bells', which we were still singing when Dr Nedungadi, the resident ayurvedic doctor, appeared, cunningly disguised as Father Christmas. The Divine Child, the one and only child in the ashram, was not the only one to leap up and hug him. The crowd, fuelled by the sound of 'Jingle Bells' on a continuous loop, went mad. The good doctor was mobbed for the contents of his sack – genuine plastic *Arati* lamps and candleholders were held high in the air as Jusep and Charlie led the *sadhus*, *swamis* and guests in a pogoing session worthy of the Sex Pistols at the Notre Dame Assembly Hall.

The crowd chanted the carol's chorus as they jumped up and down, and the *sadhu* with the dreadlocks, which usually lay in a serpent-like coil around the top of his head, suddenly pulled out the pin that had been holding everything together. The 4-ft ropes of hair created a May Pole effect and spun the Divine Child, the Swoony Swami, the American *swami*, Astrid, Cartier, Dan, Charlie, the two Ronits, Jusep and anyone else caught in its vortex, beyond the usual rules of gravity. No one was immune. Millicent's glasses misted up as she clapped and beamed. Even Ravi, normally a man with a solid attachment to the ground, was wobbling across the floor, laughing, singing and clapping his hands with glee.

We eventually came to rest an hour later, hot, sweaty and swaying, in the Dhanwantari Hall where Swami*s* Swoony and American united to cut a huge chocolate sponge cake proclaiming 'Happy Christmas' in brown and white icing.

It was quite simply the best Christmas Eve I have ever had. I went to bed feeling quite giddy, and happy that at last we had the words for the grand finale of the nativity play.

I woke up the next morning with a racing pulse and a hangover worthy of several bottles of wine. I couldn't believe I hadn't been drinking. I had slept through the fan, Millicent's snoring, Minnie Mouse's red-hot coal-walking and the gong. How the heck was I going to write the play by midday? I am afraid that those dormitory toilets were not quite as clean that day as they might have been, but I thought that, under the circumstances, God and the Swoony Swami would understand.

I almost did it. Only one hour late. I was sitting up in the Health Hut discussing the finer details of the script with Cartier and Dan over a restorative fruit salad when Astrid appeared. Could I go directly to the Shiva Hall? Charlie and all the actors, including the three wise men, were waiting for me and the script.

'You're late,' said Charlie.

'You didn't give me much time, Charlie.'

'Bloody writers,' said Charlie, not entirely jokingly.

Astrid went off to get some photocopies of the script while Cartier went to make me a cup of *chai* and Dan coached me in some cleansing *kapalabhati* breathing.

I would have to deal with Charlie later. There was too much to do, and Joseph and Mary had booked in for another massage at three.

Although I was cross with him I had to admit that Charlie did seem to know what he was doing. Within an hour he had turned a complete shambles into something that quite closely resembled a play. Mary and Joseph looked as if they might actually be in love, the girlie chat in the beauty parlour resulted in the Swoony Swami being made '*Swami* of the Month', the details of his sculpted yogic muscles eagerly examined in Cartier's copy of *Vogue*. Ravi threw himself into the production of newborn baby cries and Millicent found some orange paint with which to create an only slightly lurid labour scene. The only hitch was Dan, who seemed unable to keep his narration in line with the unfolding of the action. Charlie took him on one side and asked him to 'focus, please'. He also asked him to remove his sunglasses, or at least put them on top of his head so he could see his script properly. He improved rapidly after that and, with Mary and Joseph running only fifteen minutes late for their massage, we were able to call it a day. 'It'll be all right on the night,' we said as we patted ourselves on the back.

The play was to be the last act in the talent show so we all settled down to watch the tirelessly bouncy Astrid, as acting MC, navigate the audience through a dizzying array of talented ashramites. Paul from Birmingham, who had been rehearsing his recitation of Sufi poetry all day, stopped himself halfway through – 'that's not how Rumi intended this poem to be read' – and started again. He got a standing ovation from Charlie. Claude, a stooped Parisian in his eighties, sang a French Christmas song with a quavering voice. A deeply charismatic South African woman performed a Negro spiritual that brought tears to all our eyes, especially Cartier's. Sally danced with that Ibizan beach sexy-girly-twirly-thingy, and a Japanese man juggled. Ravi demonstrated a little-known Chinese martial art, and a Joni Mitchell lookalike sang sweet folk songs about her hometown of Alabama.

There was a break between the rest of the talent and the play. Cast and crew went outside to enjoy some cool air and discuss any last-minute concerns. There were several.

A very worried-looking Swoony Swami had already cornered Charlie: 'Have the *sadhus* been hoodwinked? Are they aware of what they are doing?'

Fortunately Charlie turned out to have the negotiating skills of Kofi Annan. He gently reassured him that he had personally taken every step to ensure that the *sadhus* knew what was going on. 'Honestly, they are fine with it,' he said. 'They understand and are happy to take part.'

The Swoony Swami, looking unconvinced, moved on to his next concern – the representation of the ashram: 'People don't come to ashrams to have babies. You must say that they have come to take shelter.'

Charlie nodded. 'No problem.'

The Swoony Swami was also concerned about the very public birthing scene: 'In India it is a very private matter.'

Charlie agreed that there would be no orange blood, that Mary would not scream in agony, and that the baby's cries would be moderate. Ravi looked very disappointed but agreed it could be done.

For a moment it looked as if the still-worried *swami* would go into a repeat loop, but Charlie, with an expansive patience that gave no betrayal of the fact that we were due on stage in thirty seconds, ran through all of the 'very reasonable concerns' and his solutions again.

With a gentle 'OM' of acquiescence, the Swoony Swami withdrew. We were on.

On the way to the stage, Cartier and I decided it wise to take out all references to the Swoony Swami's hot body and his '*Swami* of the Month' status, replacing it with an extended debate on ashram chic. This came surprisingly easily to us and the rest of the show proceeded without a hitch – until the Swoony Swami forgot to talk about *karma* yoga in his list of rules. This was supposed to have been the cue for Mary to go into labour. There was a slight pause in which Charlie, standing in the wings, looked as though he might be the one to give birth. Fortunately Mary remembered what she was there for and the contractions began. The birth turned out to be very straightforward, Mary didn't have to scream at all and there was no row with Joseph. Ravi kept his side of the bargain and Jesus emerged into the world, a quiet, well-behaved little boy, without the faintest hint of orange blood.

We moved towards the show's climax. I was holding the Star of Bethlehem and thought Charlie had instructed me to wave it from side to side but from a stationary position. He claimed afterwards that he had told me to walk with the star to the side of the stage to guide the three wise men to the baby Jesus. Whatever. They found their way to the stage as if they had been there many times before and threw themselves into their part. They were naturals – especially the dreadlocked one, whose long coils had been pinned back into place after the Christmas Eve action and were now secured with twin half-moons. This *sadhu* knew how to work an audience.

They kneeled down before Mary and, one by one, uttered their wise words, the words the universe had been waiting to hear:

'Jingle bells.'

'Jingle bells.'

'Jingle bells.'

Dan, who had remembered all of his narrative drive, moved centre stage and led the crowd in a rousing rendition of the by now very familiar carol. The *sadhus* danced in the manner of Christmas Eve while cast and crew felt the warm glow of a job well done.

~ 6 ~

'I need to be with gentle people'

Cast and crew spent Boxing Day, and several of the days that followed, exhausted but firmly bonded. The Health Hut became our unofficial clubhouse and we met there as often as we could, between *asana* practice, *satsangs*, chickpea curries and selfless actions.

We marvelled at Charlie's performance in front of the Swoony Swami.

'Charlie is a very intelligent man,' sighed Astrid.

I nodded in agreement, and the two of us sighed together.

We also marvelled at the growth of our hair and nails, and decided that the ashram food must be good for us after all. We were enjoying the *asana* practice – although it seemed to involve a bit too much standing on our heads. Astrid didn't like the arm-balancing postures either, but Cartier argued that they were great for muscle definition. Astrid agreed to persevere. Ravi liked *savasana* best.

The only place I wasn't happy was in my bedroom. Millicent's snoring could still be heard through the earplugs Cartier had given me, and frankly, well, we just weren't getting on. I felt her disapproval of my hairdrying and make-up habits – the fact that usage of both had diminished considerably under the pressure of the ashram timetable had not assuaged her fondness for calling me 'The Make-up Queen'.

Tensions reached a head one day when I got back from another muggy afternoon's *asana* practice desperate for a shower. I knew it was her turn to go first, these things having been carefully demarcated early on in the relationship, but she wasn't home, so I leapt into the ice-cold trickle with joy in my heart. The voice of disapproval soon came from beyond the bathroom door. I think calling me a 'selfish bitch' was a bit much – though I had to admit it made a welcome change from 'dear'.

The only person who didn't join us in the Health Hut was Dan. A funny thing happened at the *puja* for the Divine Mother on Boxing Day evening. Menstruating women were banned from attending, which seemed ironic given that it was a Mother we were supposed to be worshipping. I could have lied and gone anyway, but I was knackered. Astrid and Cartier decided to uphold the sisterhood and skive off with me. We sat on the roof terrace and ate cashew nuts and sesame balls. The subject under discussion was Dan. Astrid thought he was interested in me and was wondering what I thought. I explained that I found his gold lamé shorts off-putting, though I had seen him sunbathing that day in his Speedos on the roof terrace and there was definitely a large point of counterbalance.

Seeing Dan leave the ceremony, Astrid mischievously asked him to 'come up and join the girls'. But it turned out that he had just had a spiritual epiphany – no toilets involved, as with my friend Caroline, just lots of incense and *kumkum*. I wondered if there had been more than just sugar in the *prasad*, the blessed food handed out at the end of the *puja*. Whatever the cause, the transformation was immediate and complete – Dan was reborn. The 'ooh err missus' chatshow host, for whom the only point of every sentence was to bring out its latent sexual innuendo, had left the building. He sat as if in a trance, his eyes staring vacantly into the distance, and declined all our offers of sesame balls and conversation.

We saw him the next day, standing by the water cooler and gazing deeply into the eyes of a fellow ashramite. I was worried about him and tried to talk to him at dinner. He put his hands to his lips requesting that silence be observed. 'I am deepening my spiritual practice, Lucy, taking a spiritual moment,' he said. 'Please respect that.'

I laughed, thinking he was joking, but he wasn't.

Dan left the ashram two days later. He had originally been planning to fly home via Singapore to pick up some duty free electronic goodies – a digital camera, an iPod and an iMac were on his Christmas list – but I suspect that his plans might have changed. I never found out. Despite a last-ditch attempt to resurrect our friendship in the Health Hut where he told me, 'I need to be with gentle people', the Dan we had all known and loved (well, all of us except Charlie) was lost to us for ever.

We decided to put it behind us. In any case, an exciting development was soon to take our mind off things: Astrid and I were to join Cartier and Charlie in the advanced *asana* class, taught by the Swoony Swami.

Millicent had told me that Vishnu-devananda was a great teacher and 'trailed a cloud of soothing energy wherever he went'. It seemed the Swoony Swami trailed the same cloud. There were many of us in its wake. In fact, his very presence seemed to radiate peaceful vibrations. Everybody wanted to be with him, or near him, to draw on his energy and strength, to feel those vibrations.

I guess it was this magnetic power that drew me up the mountain. I can't think of any other reason why I would have gone – I hate heights. It would also be fair to say that I hadn't registered the momentous nature of this walk. I certainly hadn't realized that we would be coming back down in the dark otherwise I am sure I would have carried a torch.

It started well enough – gentle slopes, meadows and the scent of end-of-the-day flowers – but just as I was beginning to consider what else I might do that evening besides climb a mountain, the path angle began to increase at an alarming rate. In perfect symphony (some might say they were working together), the path surface also began to shift from a bed of dried mud, pebbles and petals into something altogether rockier. Eventually I was faced with a pile of rocks so big they looked fake – like misplaced extras from *Ben Hur*. Unfortunately, Charlton Heston did not choose that moment to make a steely-faced appearance, and nor did his chariot. Finally, the individual rocks joined forces and became one big rock – with no footholds. To make matters worse, the mountain was sacred so we had to walk the final distance in bare feet. The light was already beginning to fade. I took off my trainers, wondering if I would ever see them again, and ended up crawling on my hands and knees to the summit – too embarrassed to take hold of the Swoony Swami's outstretched hand.

Once there I sat petrified by fear. The Swoony Swami smiled at me kindly and promised we would go back directly after he had chanted the *Arati* Prayer, but he hadn't reckoned on the surprise *puja* that the local villagers had organized. A fire was lit and there followed worship, involving bananas and some drumming. Then there was the distribution of a delicious rice puddingy creation and a treacly liquid that tasted like mince pies, both of which had been carried up the mountain in large tin buckets by the villagers and were served piping hot on banana leaves. This wintry English food was very welcome given that the temperature had, for the first time since I'd been in India, slipped well below 30°C. Then there were some fireworks that lit up the otherwise dark valley many, many metres below. A smell of burning rubber filled the air, and I found myself worrying once again about my trainers.

Three hours later we started our descent. Cartier and Astrid took one of my arms each and the three of us, with the help of a fireman called Dave from Nebraska, put one foot in front of the other until we were delivered to the safety of the ashram gate. I am glad to report that nobody was hurt in the climbing of the mountain, but we were all a bit pissed off with Charlie, who was nowhere to be seen. Rumour had it that he and Jusep had found a natural cave about halfway down, a little off the beaten track, and had stopped for a *beedi* and some swigs from the hip flask.

The next day I went to another of the Swoony Swami's lectures. He was explaining the first two of the so-called 'eight limbs' described in Patanjali's yoga *sutras*. I was intrigued. These eight disciplines, a treatise for eliminating suffering, culminating in the attainment of *samadhi*, had proved remarkably enduring – the *sutras* were written around two thousand years ago – about the time the Romans invaded Britain – and seemed to be more relevant today than ever – providing the follower with a well of spiritual substance from which to draw in the face of the materialistic demands of twenty-first-century daily life.

The *yamas* are 'the ethical codes we try to use in our daily life as our spiritual base', the five disciplines that govern the way we behave towards other people. He wrote them on the blackboard.

Ahimsa – non-violence – applies not just to our physical actions, but also to our mental and verbal actions. Each negative thought has a triple whammy effect, he told us, 'harming the person who is thinking it, unconsciously affecting the person who is the subject of the thought and bouncing back again onto the person who thought it'.

'*Satya* means truthfulness.' The Swoony Swami looked sad. 'We are all liars, very ready to make excuses for ourselves. Our version of the truth is often self-serving.'

We all looked shamefully at our feet and were glad to move on to *aparigraha* – Dragon Man's 'possessing only what is necessary'.

The next one was *asteya*, which the Swoony Swami defined as non-stealing. 'Even talking more than we need to is a form of stealing from someone else. We must remember that we actually don't own anything, not even our own bodies, of which we are caretakers.'

'*Brahmacharya* means purity and sexual restraint.' The audience moved forward – what would the Swoony Swami say about sex? Did he have sexual thoughts? 'It's not about repression, but about raising ourselves above the instinct. The sexual instinct is actually our mind – the genitals have no instinct – so, as a thought, we should be able to control it … Sex is OK as an expression of love and to create human beings, but to waste it seeking momentary gratification is an abuse of a Divine gift.'

'Does that apply to masturbation?' asked an eager member of the audience.

'Yes. The saying "masturbation makes you blind" is probably true – spiritually, rather than physically blind.'

There were also five *niyamas*; these are the practices that help us to create a disciplined body and mind.

Saucha means purity of mind and body – eating hygienic food, regular bathing, thinking pure thoughts, keeping a clean and tidy home.

Tapas – meaning 'that which generates heat' – are acts that increase our spiritual fervour, 'like getting up at five-thirty, sitting on a hard floor, meditating for half an hour. You do it because you know it will do you good and after about six months you start to enjoy it. Every time we are successful we build our spiritual willpower.'

Svadhyaya requires us to study in order to better understand ourselves. 'If you don't have a guru you should read books about saints for inspiration.'

Santosha is contentment. The Swoony Swami urged us to be happy in ourselves, 'making a distinction between what we need and what we want. When we are in an ashram we realize that we don't need much. Living in the present, giving attention to what you have, reducing desires. This is the way of *santosha*.'

And finally '*isvara-pranidhana* – reducing the ego, surrendering to the ultimate reality – to God and Divine powers'.

I think we all felt a little overwhelmed, but the Swoony Swami said the scale of the operation shouldn't put us off. 'Just to be good in one of them would make you a saint,' he said, and quoted Swami Sivananda: '"To be able to develop one virtue in a lifetime is a great feat."'

He suggested that we start by choosing one of the virtues and noting down our thoughts in relation to it throughout the day, that 'to observe the nature of the mind, to start to become aware of it, enables us to make changes. This way we can really start to know and transform ourselves.'

Which one to choose? They all seemed so difficult – except *brahmacharya*, which I seemed to be doing pretty well, although this was not entirely of my own making. I joined the end of what had become a very long queue of people, mainly women, who wanted to talk to him in person, to ask his advice about the handling of their *yamas* and *niyamas*. I also wanted to thank him for saving me on the mountain, well, for offering me his hand anyway.

By the time I got to the front of the queue the Swoony Swami was running short of time, so we arranged to meet a little later for a proper chat in reception. Charlie kept walking in and out and winking at me, which made me cross. I glared at him. Eventually he disappeared but not before giving me the thumbs-up and another massive wink.

I hoped that the Swoony Swami hadn't noticed. I asked him if he missed his life in the West and his old career as a paediatrician. He said that he got the same pleasure out of looking after people's spiritual well-being here. 'I like to spend time with the people,' he said, 'creating the right energy, because it's the people who create the vibrations in the ashram.'

I told him that I was having a tremendous time, really enjoying the ashram's vibrations.

'Yes, Lucy, you seem really happy, you have a lightness of being.' He looked at me again. 'Your face is shining.'

I didn't like to tell him that my 'lightness of being' was intermittent at best, and generally at its lowest ebb when talking to Millicent, or that the shine would probably disappear when he left the room.

He got up. My shine did disappear. I felt shabby. With all his talk of creating the right energy in the ashram I felt especially bad that it seemed to be awash with people getting hickeys and spending long periods of time on the roof terrace under the stars. The truth, the *satya*, was that I would have been one of them if I could have found someone to exchange hickeys with. But I did really wanted to change – to stop seeing finding a man as the answer, to find a life of deeper meaning independent of anyone else. The Swoony Swami really did make me want to be a better human being. I would make a commitment to the *yamas* and *niyamas* – they were a good place to start – but eventually, when I became a real Yoga Goddess, I would have to live and breathe all 195 of those *sutras*.

To kick off this new approach to life I decided to forgive Charlie – firstly for the rude way in which he talked to me when I delivered the script just a little bit late, secondly for not helping me down the mountain and thirdly for winking at me in reception. Anyway it would be good to wipe the slate clean. He, along with Cartier and Jusep, had reached the end of their natural ashram life. Jusep was going to a full moon party in Goa; Cartier and Charlie were both going to Varkala, a beach resort a couple of hours away. Cartier needed to do some shopping and Charlie wanted to get some sand between his toes. He had to be back in London at the beginning of January to film a docu-drama featuring some porn stars.

Astrid and I were both keen to stick around the ashram for a bit longer, so we agreed to meet up again with Cartier and Charlie in a few days' time. We would have a New Year reunion on the beach. From there – well, I had a loose plan. I was keen to follow in Ben and Erik's footsteps – to go and see the Hugging Mother, affectionately known as 'Amma' or, to give her full nomenclature, 'Mata Amritanandamayi Devi', meaning 'the Divine Mother who finds bliss in the nectar of immortality'. Her ashram was just a couple of hours' drive from

Varkala. I'd read *Holy Cow* and the woman who wrote that had not only got a hug, but also the bigger boobs that she had wished for. This persuaded Astrid and Cartier to come, too. We spent several hours trying to decide what we would wish for. Charlie was a huge supporter of bigger boobs.

I threw myself into my last three days of ashram life, a whirlwind of mind-expanding activity. I attended all of Dr Nedungadi's ayurvedic lectures and uncovered some useful tips, amongst them a cure for constipation, a common ashram problem with a diet so rich in rice. 'When that little fellow won't come out,' said the doctor, 'instead of putting your hands to your forehead and straining, press the marma point on the middle of your chin and sing a good song – I suggest "Amazing Grace".'

We were also encouraged to scrape our tongues with a bitter paste called *triphala*. 'If you are doing every day there will be no sagging of the cheeks and there will be no ageing until sixty-five.'

I thought of the taxi driver's 'cheeks coming like apples' exercise – this would be a useful replacement.

There were several commercial breaks in which the good doctor unveiled the benefits of *panchakarma* – 'sends the toxins out, isn't it?' – and the 400-rupee massage during which the ageing process would be checked, fatigue prevented, eyesight improved, the lustre of the skin polished, the mind and body rejuvenated, and the body brought to perfect health.

The evening cultural programme continued at a blistering pace. Kalaripayattu martial artists from Kochi played with fire. A 'Jesus Travels' bus brought beautiful young girls from the Gayathri School to perform a classical Bharatanatyam dance with bells on their feet and brilliant red dots in the centre of their palms. There was much exaggeration of eye movements, finger-flicking and golden head-dress bling

bling. There was also an evening of *santoor* music into which Sri Haridas, an honoured master of the '100-stringed lute', urged us to delve more deeply: 'This was just a drop in the great ocean of Indian classical music. Please drink from the nectar of Indian music. We wish you a very melodious New Year.'

With all this stimulation it was hardly surprising that my hair grew another inch. In fact, I was feeling great all over. The ashram's unofficial detox programme – no stimulants, five hours of yoga a day, extreme mountain walking – rivalled the Betty Ford Clinic, but at a fraction of the price. It had been hard to start with but it had been worth it. My body felt stronger, I had gained some muscle definition and I'd dropped several years on the massage table, a massage so thorough that the only thing that didn't get a good going over were the bits of me safely tucked away inside. Even my co-ordination had improved. I learned to eat without spraying myself, or my neighbours, with chickpea curry, and my taste buds mellowed sufficiently to be able to distinguish one vegetable from another.

John decided that it was time for a selfless action promotion and I began a new career as an ashram tea lady, helping Astrid bring four huge tin teapots to the thirsty crowds twice a day. Astrid did the sweet tea and I did 'no sugar'. Together we got to know our customers' preferences: some liked big cups; the Swoony Swami took a small one; Millicent aimed for three cups of unsweetened and complained bitterly when we ran out; the Germans told me, on a daily basis, that there was not enough unsweetened tea. Did they think I had shit for brains? I knew all about the laws of supply and demand – it was one of the things a career in advertising had taught me. The problem lay in the dark recesses of the kitchen where there was a complete incomprehension that anyone could like something that wasn't sweet. One day I got the man in charge to promise he would make an extra pot of unsweetened tea at lunchtime – a fact I announced to all my customers at breakfast time – but he had an argument with his wife in the course of the morning and forgot his promise. At lunchtime there was only sweet tea – or sweet tea. I forgave him but the baying crowd were not so lenient with me. Tensions were at bursting point when a German girl tried to pull a full pot of scalding sweet tea out of my hand. Fortunately it was only the lid that clattered to the floor but I was able to use the opportunity to say 'enough is enough' and do things my way for the rest of the tea break. I went back to my room to contemplate my progress in *ahimsa*, the non-violence *yama*. Exactly how far had I developed my ability to restrain those physical, mental and verbal actions? And, come to think of it, how much headway had my fellow students made along the path to the non-covetous state of *aparigraha*?

I always hoped that the Swoony Swami would see me working hard – walking tirelessly back and forth from the kitchen to the Dhanwantari Hall where the tea was served – but the only authority figure I encountered was a woman who told me off for wearing a T-shirt that apparently didn't provide enough coverage of my navel. I asked her to bear with me until I could put the two huge pots of tea down safely in the Hall but she was having none of it. I had to stop and make the half a centimetre adjustment there and then.

And suddenly it was time to leave. New Year's Eve morning dawned and Astrid and I joined the silent walk down to the lake. The cadets were not with us this time, but the locals were out and about performing their morning rituals, and jumping on their cow's back to give it a good scrub behind the ears.

I looked over at the Swoony Swami. He seemed so peaceful, vibrating gently in the early morning sun. I was tempted to stay longer. Walking the *yama* and *niyama* path would probably be easier here than in the outside world and there was no doubt that ashram life had been good for me – physically and mentally. I'd had one of the happiest Christmases ever and made some good friends. It had all been so much fun. It didn't feel as I imagined a spiritual journey should feel – there had been no austerities, but then, on the downside, there had been no obvious epiphanies either. In fact, the main spiritual attraction had been the Swoony Swami. Could I become one of his sunbeams on a more long-term basis? Hmm. I seemed to have done that clichéd Western thing of falling for my spiritual leader.

But I had the feeling that the reality of life as an ashram resident would be a very different thing to the spiritual entertainment camp we had been enjoying. Ultimately, ashram life was supposed to involve the giving up of worldly pleasures, wasn't it? And when it came down to it, did I really want to dedicate my life to making the ashram tea? And really I couldn't stand Millicent's snoring any more, not even for another night. She had also developed the unappealing habit of curtailing my use of the hairdryer by switching off the master electricity switch outside our room door and pretending it was a power cut. I was also worried by a conversation with my father on Christmas Day when he had accused me of sounding pious regarding my lack of alcohol intake. It was no good. I couldn't let my family down like this – I had to go and have a drink. It was New Year's Eve after all.

New Year's Eve in Varkala turned out to be a low-key affair. I'd spent the afternoon mooning about, missing the ashram and the Swoony Swami, first on the beach watching the eagles soaring high up in the thermals, then in the bunting-strewn cafés which lined the narrow pathway above the red cliffs of Varkala, and finally in the Tibetan shops with Cartier, my newly appointed personal stylist. But nothing, not even a turquoise shoulder bag, could lift my mood. We spent the evening at the Brown Indian, a laidback café serving rum and cola concealed in teapots, contemplating the moonlit sea far beneath us and eating Parmesan cheese and fresh olives, thoughtfully brought by an Italian ashramite's wife who had arrived that morning from Rome. At midnight the couple cracked open several bottles of Veuve Cliquot and we toasted the Swoony Swami and Charlie.

Charlie had attended an ayurvedic cooking course the day before we'd arrived and had been overcome with enthusiasm for his efforts, and those of his fellow classmates. As if this wasn't enough, when the instructor had suggested he should include lots of molasses and honey in his diet to soothe the fiery heat of an overactive *pitta* constitution, Charlie had rushed to the nearest roadside stall and overdosed on syrupy rosogulla balls, which had been heated by the sun over the course of several days. Whichever was the root cause of Charlie's problems, the results were the same: an even more fiery constitution, a temperature of 104 degrees and a very pressing need to be in close proximity to a toilet.

I woke up on New Year's Day morning full of hungover regret. If I had stayed at the ashram I might have been merging with cosmic bliss rather than wondering where my paracetamol were. I switched on my phone and wiped my eyes, which were still caked in smeary kohl. In amongst the flurry of New Year text messages from ever more pissed friends and relatives was one from Charlie. He was also in need of drugs: 'Lucy, am poorly sick. Bring paracetamol and water. Please hurry.'

The text had been sent at 5 a.m. It was now eleven. Shit. Memories of Mysore and the pomegranates were still fresh enough in my mind – I knew how this could go. There was no time to waste. Cartier, Astrid and I jumped in a rickshaw, picked up all of the antibiotics we could find and hurtled round to Charlie's guesthouse. He was still alive. Fortunately his landlady had been a little more attentive than us and had taken him to the hospital for a fever-reducing injection. We spent the next three days doing penance – taking it in turns to mop his brow, replenish his drinking water and change the CDs on his Walkman. 'Charlie's Angels' were born.

A gentle trip up the backwaters in a houseboat seemed to be the perfect convalescence. As soon as he was well enough, we packed Charlie and ourselves into an Ambassador and bounced off to

Alappuzha to collect the crew and a boat. Our spirits soon revived, especially as the driver had a Kylie CD that contained the highly appropriate 'Fever'. The three Angels hitched their sarongs high in imitation of Kylie's nurse uniform and conducted a perfectly hand-choreographed rendition of the video that had brought a smile to the face of many a man. Charlie beamed appreciatively and suggested we might all like to go to his fortieth birthday party to be held that summer in the south of Spain. We agreed.

Our high spirits tumbled at the sight of our boat – more council house than Beckingham Palace. The photos we had been shown by our travel agent in Varkala had portrayed a relaxed world of wicker sun loungers, white daybeds and smiling uniformed staff serving highballs on silver trays. Our boat was covered in blue tarpaulin, a mattress lay gypsy-like out front and plastic white chairs were to be our loungers. Our staff consisted of one young lad and two toothless old men dressed in checked *lungis* drawn up to the knees and dirty shirts, except Harish who was proudly sporting a 'Ray-Ban Made in USA' T-shirt. There was no alcohol but they offered to go and buy us some Kingfisher and Sprite when we docked at lunchtime – if we gave them the money.

We tried ringing our man back in Varkala but he was suddenly unable to speak English. All of the other boats were apparently fully booked. There was nothing for it but to put up and shut up. Actually, as soon as we left the harbour, we began to calm down. Charlie had discovered that Cartier was a highly talented roller of spliffs and set her to work on a production line that eventually spanned the entire length of the white plastic table.

The Angels spent the afternoon sunbathing on the gypsy mattress while Charlie captained the ship, his convalescing head shaded from the sun by Harish, the proud owner of a black umbrella. Charlie steered our way through the plant life, as Pradeep, the ship's boy, risked his limbs trying to separate the more persistent weeds from around the motor – as it was running. Charlie cut a really quite skilful path through the crisscrossing *vallams*, the traditional dugouts which ferried passengers, shaded by the ubiquitous black umbrella, back and forth across the water. Children floated in old tyres and dive-bombed each other from the palm-lined banks. These trees camouflaged a hive of activity – coir-making, washing days, rice-growing and importantly 'toddy-tapping'. Charlie persuaded Harish to stop and let us buy some toddy – traditional fermented coconut juice. It tasted fizzy and revolting, but the crew seemed to like it so we gave it to them along with a bottle of the Kingfisher they had gone off to get us at lunchtime. We spent the rest of the afternoon and evening getting very, very stoned.

I would like to claim that we spent the evening reading the diaries of the famous Indian poet, Rabindranath Tagore, who had a spiritual experience in his houseboat when it was flooded by the light of the moon. Unfortunately, I have little recollection of the evening beyond playing 'Shoot, Shag or Marry', in which opinion was divided over who to shoot, but all the girls wanted to shag Jusep and marry the Swoony Swami. Charlie wanted to shag one Ronit and marry the other.

I ended up in bed with Charlie. I know this because I woke up there and because I have some memory of reading each other extracts from Hermann Hesse's *Siddhartha* until late in the night. But judging by the conversation in the Ambassador the next morning, in which Charlie spoke at some length about his Internet dating experiences and how gorgeous Israeli girls are, we were still firmly located in the friendship zone. Shame. The truth was, I could quite happily have shot, shagged and married him, all at the same time.

~7~

'Durga, Durga, Durga'

The two-hour car ride to the Hugging Mother was a rather more subdued affair than the journey to the houseboat; we were all nursing very bad hangovers – so bad in fact that the experience of the sun rising on yet another beautiful Keralan day was a painful one.

We arrived in the tiny hamlet of Vallikkavu, populated only by waiting taxi drivers, and took a small ferryboat across the river, punted by a man as long and thin and brown as his pole. The first we saw of the ashram were two pink tower blocks that rose gaudily out of the lush green coconut groves. The second thing we saw was a fellow Sivananda ashramite, Cath. We bumped into her at the ashram pier. She looked pale and thin, a shadow of the happy-go-lucky girl we had last seen two days ago bouncing around the Brown Indian with a glass of Veuve Cliquot in her hand.

'I've got to get out of here,' she said firmly. 'I feel like shit.'

'Do you think you ate something funny?' I asked – I was beginning to be able to spot the signs.

'No, it's this place. I feel totally drained; all the devotees are so miserable – so pale and thin, they won't even look you in the eye. It's like – can't get a shag get a hug.'

'Did you get your hug?' asked Astrid with concern.

Cath looked miserable. 'Yes, but I didn't feel anything.'

We tried to get her to come and have a cup of *chai* with us but she couldn't be persuaded.

'Sorry – just got to go. Keep in touch. Bye.'

And with that she picked up her rucksack and jumped on the ferry-boat, which was just about to return to the other side.

We looked at each other. Something must have happened – she wasn't telling us the whole story. How could one night with a Hugging Mother affect a person so badly?

Charlie, who was in a hurry because he had to get back to London to start organizing the porn star shoot, decided to join the afternoon express hugging queue, reportedly the same quality of hug as the evening session but without the trimmings. He would leave straight afterwards. He headed off towards a large pink temple – guarded by two red velvet umbrellas with gold tassels and a team of five plaster horses drawing wildly coloured deities behind them. Astrid, Cartier and I decided that we weren't going to let Cath's demeanour influence us – we would join the evening ceremony as planned, and stay overnight.

'*Darshan*' – the giving of an audience by a master – took place four nights a week at Amma's ashram, but Sunday was the big one. This was *Devi Bhava Darshan* and 20,000 visitors were expected to join the ashram's 2,500 permanent residents in witnessing Amma enter '*Bhava*' – a state of high emotion in which she would completely forget herself and merge with her beloved namesake Devi, or Divine Mother. This would be *Bhakti* yoga, the yoga of love and devotion, at its finest.

Consequently the ashram was very busy. White-faced, white-robed, shorn-headed devotees hurried by, their singularity, pace and monochromatic appearance in stark contrast to the families of hirsute, colourful Indians who promenaded slowly up and down the heat bowl of the sand-filled courtyard. Small boys stood stiffly in unfamiliar suits, while their little sisters, eyes lined with kohl and ears heavy with gold rings, hid their primrose-yellow sparkly nylon dresses with matching hair and shoe bows in the folds of their mother's Sunday best sari.

Amma was everywhere. Her round face, the smiling innocent face of a child, betraying none of its fifty years, beamed down from key rings, tapes and endless photos at the souvenir stalls in the courtyard, and again on the 'Chant Your *Mantra*' and 'Be Innocent' stickers sold in the official gift shop. There was even a room selling Amma dolls made by the ashram's residents. In all representations, whatever their form, she was the picture of perfect health and youthful vitality – her eyes, hair and skin shone, the broad smile revealed perfect Hollywood teeth, and something truly nasty in me was pleased to see that the diamond in her nose stud was so much bigger than Shanti's, so much more bling.

While Astrid stood in the registration line with our passports, Cartier and I cruised the wall notices around the upstairs balcony of the pink temple. One notice proclaimed: '"In this age of selfishness, self-less service is the only soap that purifies". Amma requests everyone to give two hours of selfless service daily.' Amma was clearly a devoted selfless server. The articles on the noticeboards revealed a vast network of charitable activities for which she had received many honours, among them the Ghandi-King Award for Non-Violence, at the presen-tation of which it was said that 'she stands here in front of us, God's love in a human body'.

Cartier had picked up the January issue of the Indian women's monthly *Savvy* magazine, on the cover of which Amma made an unlikely star alongside 'Bride in Waiting' and Bollywood actress Raveena Tandon. She'd read that Amma chairs a business empire worth £250 million with plans for a commercial TV channel and business partnerships with multi-national corporations – hardly surprising then that senior government officials were falling over themselves to support the ashram's activities. 'This woman,' Cartier had said, holding up the double-page feature with the headline 'Godwoman or brandmaker?' for Astrid and me to see, 'is smart.'

A lot of money had been spent on building the town that the Amritapuri Ashram had become. There were the two bright pink, brand-new accommodation tower blocks for visitors and long-term residents, rooms for those living the celibate life of *brahmacharya*, hostels for the ashram's student population, kitchens, shops, offices, AmritaNet, a travel desk, two libraries, a swimming pool, a beach, a cowshed, a refuge for two baby elephants, two canteens – one Western and one Indian – and the largest *darshan* hall in southern India. At 30,000 sq ft and no get-in-the-way pillars, the 20,000 who regularly attended the *Devi Bhava* would have plenty of room to swing their 108 *mala* meditation beads.

Very little money had been spent on the decor of our bedroom. It was spartan in the extreme. 'At least it's clean,' said Astrid brightly, 'and at least we don't have to share it with anyone else.' That was true. With the three brown plastic mattresses down on the tiled floor there was little room for our rucksacks and suitcases, let alone another person. 'And at least there's a great view,' added Astrid, pointing at the canopy of palm trees that stretched for miles into the distance, interrupted only by our pink sister tower block.

Coming back down from the fifteenth floor we bumped into Charlie. The hug had happened quickly; there had only been a few people in the queue and the Hug Stewards were in a no-nonsense mood. Charlie had enjoyed it but he said it was no different to the hug he might get from someone in the street.

'And, then what happened?'

'Well, that was it. Oh, and she whispered something in my ear – sounded like "truck, truck, truck" – and I felt quite hot, but that was all.'

We were disappointed.

'What did you wish for Charlie?' asked Astrid.

'Nothing, I forgot,' he said, ruefully.

It was time to say goodbye to Charlie. His hug was strong and made me feel quite hot, but I was glad that he left quickly. I was sad to see him go. Despite our differences I had become fond of him over the last couple of weeks and would have liked to travel together a while longer, but he had to get back to London and apply himself to the recruitment of porn stars. I joined the others sitting on the ledge by the *chai* stall, sandwiched between two halves of an Indian family. We sat in silence for several minutes contemplating our new Charlie-less status. Without Charlie, well, we weren't Angels any more, were we? It felt very strange to be without our wings.

A slice of pizza at the Western Café soon cheered us up, despite the fierce looks of the white-robed and white-faced. Melinda was also white-robed but there the similarity ended. She had the excitable, corkscrew black curls and blue, sparkling eyes of a ten-year-old, although she told us later that she was fifty-three. She beckoned us over with a big smile and this hair, which sprung out of her scalp with great exuberance, as if it could be contained no longer. I couldn't take my eyes off it; I swear I could see it growing.

'Why is everyone so miserable here?' I wondered aloud.

'Oh, take no notice. Ashram politics. People who have been here too long and are too caught up in the power struggles – trying to get close to Amma. It's a difficult energy to be around – I couldn't live here.'

Melinda had received her first hug in her hometown of Sydney on one of Amma's world tours. She turned out to be the font of all knowledge.

'Why does she hug so many people?' I asked.

'Amma is the embodiment of unconditional love. She says that her only wish is to spend her whole life with her hand on someone's shoulder, consoling them, holding them to her heart and wiping away their tears, until her dying breath. She has embraced more than twenty million people around the world – she is tireless, never stops; an amazing woman.'

'I read that she even hugged a leper,' said Cartier, wincing.

'Yes, he came to her with caterpillar-like sores that hung off every inch of his body. Everyone was feeling sick at the sight of him. Her devotees wanted to send him away but she had him brought to her and she actually licked the pus oozing from the sores. She nursed his wounds for six months until he was healed.'

We joined Cartier in a chorus of 'Eeuwww'.

Melinda smiled. 'I know it's hard to understand, but she regards everyone, even the prime minister of this country, as her children.'

'And how many children does she have?' asked Astrid, happily embracing a change of subject.

'Oh no, Amma is not a biological mother – actually she has never even had a period. She has a blood test every six months and technically she should be dead – she has every disease under the sun.'

I was slightly going off the idea of having a hug, and I could see Cartier was, too.

Melinda saw our faces and laughed. 'Don't worry. Amma can't be judged by our standards – she is not a human being in the normal sense of the word. Even as a child it was obvious that she was quite different. Her mother had no labour pains giving birth and she came into the world beaming from ear to ear, and with this funny dark-blue complexion – the complexion of Lord Krishna. By the age of five she was composing devotional songs and going off into the woods to meditate.'

'What did her mother think of all this?' I asked.

'Oh, the family were completely freaked by her meditations, chanting and singing. They mistook the constant moving of her lips for madness – when in fact she was just praying silently. They stopped her schooling and she became the family servant. But this didn't stop her. She sang as she worked, slipped into reveries and took the family food to feed the village Untouchables. It was only when she started to attract the attention of the outside world that they understood that she was Self-Realized. Then they allowed her to hold *darshan* in one half of the family cowshed. The cowshed is still here, though Amma couldn't fit all her followers in there any more.'

Melinda's hair grew another inch, and her eyes twinkled. She clearly regarded Amma as a living saint, and wanted us to feel the same way.

'You know, because you're first-timers you girls could go up on stage tonight and sit with Amma. And if you behave yourselves you might be allowed to join the *Prasad* Queue.'

'The *Prasad* Queue?' asked Cartier. (She didn't do queues.)

'Yes, it's a great honour, only for Westerners,' said Melinda warmly. 'You hand Amma the *prasad* – paper-wrapped bundles of sweets – and she gives them to her devotees.'

Cartier decided that, just for today, she did do queues.

We selflessly made chapattis for an hour, trying not to be discouraged by the scowling faces of the white-faced and white-robed, and then rushed back to our room for cold showers and wardrobe dilemmas. By the time we made our way down to the huge hall in our finest white *darshan* dresses, Amma was already in full swing, sitting centre-stage, robed in white and surrounded by men in orange. Musicians and chanters sat in front of her, at the foot of the stage. Everyone was singing *bhajans* accompanied by *tablas* and harmoniums. Women sat on the right of the hall, men to the left. We joined the sisterhood, alternately clapping, OM'ing and shuffling forwards to accommodate another set of Indian mothers, aunties, grannies and granddaughters. Every so often Amma's arms would flare up – perhaps a sign that she was moving closer to that state of emotional ecstasy in which she would feel at one with her beloved Devi. Her pace was slow, trance-like, her eyes shut. She already looked exhausted, even though it was only seven o'clock.

She left the stage an hour later and then the wait began, to get a hugging time. We queued for more than an hour as the white-faced, white-robed women in charge tensely discussed the politics of *mantra* acquisition – should people who wanted a *mantra* from Amma as well as a hug queue in a different place to the people who just wanted a hug? The queues divided and reformed several times in response to their changes of mind. Suspected queue-jumpers were first of all subjected to a whispering campaign and then confronted. Tempers flared. Just as a fight was about to break out we got our hugging slot. Eleven o'clock. Some of the lollipops that signified the start of waiting lines were displaying numbers that wouldn't be reached until four or five in the morning. We noticed that there were few Western faces in these lines. Did being Western entitle us to a shorter wait as well as *prasad* bearing? Apparently so. The divisions between East and West ran deep in the ashram – different prices for food, different eating places, different work. Although Western visitors were on an embarrassingly cushy number, the Western residents didn't have it easy. On the contrary, the white-faced and white-robed worked very hard – stuffing envelopes, making pizza and pounding dough the colour of their faces into chapattis. Melinda had explained that they needed to work harder than the Indians because they had more ego to deal with. This was probably true but it wasn't doing anything to improve the mood of the white-faced and white-robed, and surely giving Western visitors earlier times and *prasad*-bearing duties would only massage these already inflated egos?

Amma reappeared an hour later. This time she sat resplendent on a throne beneath a green and gold silk umbrella. She wore a silk sari that matched the umbrella, set off with a thick, gladiator-style gold belt. Her long, black, wavy hair was swept into a neat ponytail beneath a golden crown. We sat on the floor of the hall for a while – watching the early crowd get their hug. Men and women were in separate queues coming from either end of the stage but it was hard to see much beyond this – there were so many people up there and most of them had their backs to us. We got the occasional glimpse of Amma's crown as it bobbed up and down, but we would have to wait until we got on stage before we got a better view. We moved up onto the stage and settled down at the back, craning our necks to watch the relentless queues inching forward. Now that I could see their faces, what struck me hardest was their desperation. Many of them were very poor, needy people – with little more than the clothes on their back – but they had still managed to find a bowl of fruit, or even a single apple, to give to their beloved Amma.

The women were often in tears. It was heartbreaking to watch these bird-like, dark-skinned creatures, impeccable in their best saris, frangipani braids in oil-slicked hair, women who carried entire fields on their heads, pleading with Amma in strangled voices and being manhandled away, arms outstretched, gasping for another moment with their beloved. The men seemed more in control of themselves, and determined to take their time. Amma took it all in good spirits. One man told a story that went on for several minutes and made Amma crease up laughing. It took several helpers to persuade him that his time was up. Another spoke at length in a low voice, pressing his lips to her ear, as she nodded and sighed and rubbed his back.

There were many ways to buy extra Amma time – some had brought photos for her to bless, others brought letters or garlands of marigolds, which they attempted to drape around their beloved, but which were quickly whisked away by the well-oiled backstage machine. The best ploy was to bring a necklace and ask her to tie it round your neck – this inevitably took ages; and while Amma fiddled with the cheap clasp, you remained buried in her arms.

Although the hall was big the stage was not – well, not when Amma and her throne took up the front half and the queues of hopeful huggers took up the sides. The back of the stage had to accommodate the ever-growing numbers of fruit baskets and garlands of marigolds along with the *prasad* production line, several hundred devotees allowed in on the First Timer ticket, and three ex-Angels eager to join the *Prasad* Queue.

Clearly the available space had to be carefully managed. The woman whose job this was, 'She Who Must Be Obeyed', was the epitome of haute couture elegance – fluffy white hair, a huge diamond rock of a ring and a fine white sari with gold embroidery that was definitely a cut above the usual ashram kit. Under her watchful eye and careful instruction, the helpers, older Western men and women (the younger ones all seemed to be hard at it making pizza in the Western canteen), shifted the human cargo around the stage. Devotees who had overstayed their welcome were asked to leave, politely at first, and then physically removed if this didn't work. The *Prasad* Queue was kept under an especially strict eye – queue-hopping was not tolerated. We progressed slowly from the back to the front under the very strictest of supervision: 'Stop'; 'Move into this space'; 'No, wait here a moment'; 'OK, now go'.

And finally, there we were at the front, being coached in the delicate art of *prasad*-bearing. We were to use only our right forefingers to pass Amma the paper-wrapped bundles, so that she could receive them flat into her left palm and give one each to the huggees. Then it was my turn. The whole of Amma World was resting on my trembling forefingers – I definitely didn't want to mess up. I was given nine bundles and passed on three as directed. So far so good. I looked up to see the first of these find its way into the hands of an Indian woman who was completely overcome, sobbing uncontrollably and offering Amma an entire harvest of lemons. Things got a bit sticky for a moment when, still transfixed by the lemons, which were now making their way to the back of the stage, I didn't notice that two more people had been hugged and Amma's hand was waiting for the second batch of three. I received a sharp dig in my ribs from the devotee in charge of *prasad*-bearing, and sprang back into action. After that little shock I deemed it safest to look only at Amma's hand until I had finished my duty. I did, however, manage to squeeze in a quick look at the two devotees in pole position next to Amma – one was massaging her thighs, whilst the other applied cold compresses; Amma got no exercise during her hugging marathons and apparently suffered badly from cramps. She didn't even get up to go to the loo. Perhaps she really was, as Melinda said, superhuman, or perhaps it was because she wasn't drinking any water.

Astrid and Cartier took their turn at *prasad*-bearing and tears sprang to my eyes, as if watching my two sisters getting married. Then it was time to have our hugs – I'd almost forgotten about this, my own bit of bliss, in all the excitement and heartbreak of watching other people getting theirs.

We joined the queue and inched slowly forward. In a moment it would be my turn, in a moment, in a moment … and suddenly I found myself thrown to the ground by a zealous devotee. My left hand was clamped to the floor and my head pushed down and bowed forward. Amma's left arm rested on my shoulder as she listened to a talkative young man burbling urgently away in Malayalam, the local language. Amma was all ears and kept drawing the young man to her ample bosom with her other hand. Eventually it was my turn. She drew me close, pulling my head into the stifling folds of her sari. She said, 'Durga, Durga, Durga' into my ear in an urgent, loud and ferociously hot whisper that sent heat bumps down my neck as I gasped for oxygen. I thanked her for my *prasad* and asked her for the ticket that would entitle me to go back at the end of the *darshan* for my *mantra* but she looked at me blankly – she spoke only Malayalam, and I spoke only English. There was an awkward pause. Next thing I knew, just as I realized that I had forgotten to wish for anything, I was pulled back and lifted into an upright position. The devotees went into a huddle to decide whether I could have the ticket. Cartier was already in Amma's arms and Astrid was pinned to the floor waiting her turn. I didn't register much again until the three of us somehow found our way to the ledge by the now deserted *chai* stall. We were all clutching our *mantra* tickets.

We felt dazed, confused and a little hot. We'd enjoyed our hugs but none of us had experienced flashes of blinding light. Astrid and Cartier had both made wishes – they weren't telling me what for but I bet I could have guessed. Amma had whispered 'Devi', the name of the Divine Mother herself, into Astrid's ear but Cartier, like Charlie, hadn't been able to make her deity out. I asked Melinda, who was passing by, what 'Durga' meant.

'Wow, she called you that? Amazing. Durga is an extremely beautiful and full of rage Goddess – she has a golden body, rides a lion and has ten arms in which she carries her weapons, jewels and rosaries of beads. She annihilated entire armies with tridents, arrows and swords; she was a fierce, virginal warrior. Go girl!'

Melinda's hair grew another inch in delight. Cartier and Astrid clapped and whooped. I hadn't made a wish so my boobs were no bigger but, on balance, I felt awesome.

We went back to the *darshan* hall at seven in the morning, but Amma was still hugging and wouldn't be giving out *mantras* until eleven. The hall had emptied out – there were only a few hundred left in the queue – and the atmosphere had changed from one of feverish excitement to exhaustion.

We ate at the Indian-run breakfast stall in the courtyard.

'Is anyone else tired?' said Astrid, yawning into her breakfast of *iddlies* and samba.

I was also feeling drained, and Cartier, usually the epitome of bright-eyed chic, looked tired and dirty. When two huge spoons of sugar in our *chai* didn't raise our game we began to worry. I felt as I did when I had glandular fever at eighteen – totally floored, unable to raise any energy, even to smile. We realized that we must feel just like Cath did yesterday. We looked around – nobody looked any happier for their hug. Amma might work like a Trojan, and have superhuman powers, but even she couldn't fill the bottomless pit of need that existed here. Whilst the Sivananda Ashram had been a highly enjoyable spiritual entertainment camp for stressed-out Westerners in search of some yogic

R&R, Amma's ashram seemed to me to have a very different function – providing love and hope to the desolate poor and emotionally needy. Just being around this amount of neediness was exhausting, let alone living here. No wonder the devotees looked so pale and beaten.

We were too tired to stand in another queue for our *mantras*. We waited until the office opened at nine to reclaim our passports, dragged our sorry arses into the ferryboat, took one last look at the twin pink towers and turned our backs on the ashram.

We fell into an Ambassador and slept all the way to Kochi, three hours' drive away. Cartier and I slept for the rest of the afternoon in a cheap, triple-bedded guesthouse room while Astrid, whose energy levels were back to their normal high, killed all the mosquitoes in our bathroom and went off to cycle around Jew Town. She returned to tell us about falling off her bike, the synagogue with the Chinese-porcelain-tiled floor, the clock tower, the antique shops and the smells of the spices – cinnamon, cardamom, pepper – that wafted from the spice auction rooms, and her plans to help the fishermen haul up the nets early the next day.

She'd met Jack, a yoga teacher cum painter and decorator from County Antrim, at the railway station as she was buying her train ticket for Goa. She'd accepted Jack's invitation to dinner and he seemed only slightly put out that Cartier and I turned up, too. We circled a delicious plateful of chips, barracuda and prawns at Europa, a beachside restaurant a couple of feet from the haunting sight of the preying-mantis-style, cantilevered fisherman's nets where Astrid would be working at dawn the next day. Jack had been to Amma's, and he wasn't surprised by our experience.

'Ah,' he said, taking another sip of 'tea' from the pot beneath the table, 'it's pretty obvious to me. I think Amma is operating an international energy exchange; she takes from Westerners rich in energy and gives it to the poor. A sort of spiritual Robin Hood. But don't get too upset about it – you could obviously afford it, otherwise she wouldn't have done it. You feel better now, don't you?' We agreed that we did. 'Well then.' He filled our teacups. 'Here's to Devi, Durga and um …?'

'Cartier,' said Cartier firmly.

I was going to miss these girls. Cartier left early the next morning for a flight back to New York, talking deliriously about a reunion with her washing machine and cappuccino-maker. Astrid and I had one last breakfast together. She was tired, having got up at dawn to work those fishermen's nets, but she was looking forward to a reunion with Jusep at a Goan full moon party. I'd decided that I needed a change of pace, something completely different.

There had been no further word from Richard – I assumed that he was making wedding plans, or was too stoned to send an email. Whatever, he was history. Still, no need to throw the baby out with the bathwater. I was going to fly up to Pune for a bit of input from his 'Sex Guru' – Osho. As Richard told me, Osho, a left-handed *Tantric*, believed that sex could be one of the paths to awaken the body's dormant spiritual potency. Opening the wheels of vital energy – the *chakras* – would release the vast store of untapped vital energy, the *kundalini Shakti,* from its place at the base of the spine, allowing it to flow freely up to the thousand-petalled *sahasra padma chakra* at the crown, the one that Shanti was opening with the violet vibrations of her shawl. By opening this *chakra*, I would feel all differences between myself and other beings disappear and I would transcend the limits of my physical body. Richard had explained, as we sat by Cat and Ted's swimming pool, that boundaries would disappear; all energies, all colours, sounds, matter and spirit, feelings and thoughts would converge into the bigger whole, and I would merge with cosmic bliss. Well, whether I reached these giddy heights or not, *Tantra's* emphasis on physical well-being sounded like the perfect antidote to Amma's exhausting yoga of devotion.

~ 8 ~

'Get juicy'

Opening the gate to my *chakras* would just have to wait another two hours. The maroon-clad guardsman perched on a high chair explained politely but firmly that the huge wooden gates studded with gold platelets were locked for the duration of the Brotherhood of the White Robes meeting and wouldn't open again until 8.30 p.m.

I was really tired. I'd eschewed a comfortable ride in an air-conditioned car along the three-hour Mumbai–Pune expressway in favour of riding by bus across Mumbai, from the airport to Dadar train station, and then travelling for five hours in a General Class carriage to Pune, squashed in with approximately twenty-five men, some above me on luggage racks, and the rest next to me on wooden benches. It was not an auspicious start to the promotion of *Tantric* well-being – half of the men had coughs worthy of a TB ward, and the onboard temperature must have been 40°C. But at least the total cost of the journey was only

55 rupees; a car would have been a hundred times that. The savings would pay for the first two nights at the luxurious Osho Guesthouse.

The place wasn't quite what I'd expected. I had somehow thought it would be abuzz with the sound of noisily erupting *chakras* and whoops of joy at the disappearance of boundaries and the appearance of violet vibrations. But the tree-lined road was deserted and for the first time since I'd been in India there was complete silence. Quite a relief after the rigours of the packed railway carriage, but very odd. I was just trying to make out the details of the shadowy figure in the high chair guarding the opposite gate, across the road, when Gita the Guest Greeter arrived. With no more than a nod to the guard she whisked me through that eastern gate and into a different world – as if I'd just stepped through a portal in a science fiction film. The temperature dropped at least 10°C. There were no wandering cows, no insistent horns, no pollution and no crowds. Guided by walkways so clean you could have used them to prepare a baby's bottle, we passed a 2-metre marble Buddha contemplating his navel on a rock beneath a huge tree, and lots of tables beneath maroon umbrellas.

Gita pointed at the Osho Auditorium, a huge black pyramid surrounded by a black pool of completely still water. 'The Beloveds are all inside for the "Brotherhood of the White Robes",' she said in reverential tones, 'but you cannot join the Buddhafield this evening – you need to have an HIV test and register with the office, which is closed until tomorrow morning. To share the Buddhafield's energy you must wear maroon robes during the day and white for the evening meetings, but you can wear your own clothes after the Brotherhood – so you will be OK tonight if you just stay in your room until the meeting has finished. Then you can come and get something to eat. The food here is very good.' She motioned towards an enormous area of gleaming sinks and state-of-the-art culinary equipment, lit up like an installation at The Tate. 'India's most advanced kitchen,' she said with pride.

Gita gave me some final instructions concerning the welcome tour the next day and left me to the joys of the guesthouse, which was next door to the kitchen in a tree-laden private corner. It more than lived up to my expectations. The lobby was like something out of *Architectural Digest* – spotless and silent, the epitome of understated chic. Cartier would have loved the cream floor, the Mies van der Rohe Barcelona chair in tan leather supported by silver curved slats, the matching stool, the glass coffee table, the square marble pillars, the single row of hardback books and the handsome, manicured receptionist.

My bedroom was a continuation of the theme – purified air embraced a deep-tan leather armchair, Himalayan mineral water (the most exclusive of the bottled waters), several tasteful prints and, most gloriously of all, a big double bed with a sprung mattress and Egyptian cotton sheets. The bed mesmerized me. I sat in the tan armchair and just stared at the arrangement of cream and brown cushions, which was so effusive that I would have to send out an advance search party for my pyjamas if I was to stand any chance of sliding between my sheets before 1 a.m. No TV, phone or stereo, but heck, for a girl that had spent the last few weeks on inch-thick mattresses, this was luxury living.

Feeling much improved after a long, hot shower, the first in three weeks, I went in search of some white-robed company at the Meera Café.

Tonight the self-service kitchen was offering a handsome array of beautiful people and a choice of Erbazzone, Broccoli Aglio e Olio, Bhopali Mixed Vegetables and Peshwari Chole, or brown rice and vegetables. And most of it was organic. OK, so it was more than double the price of Amma's *iddlies* and samba, but you got a free knife and fork, sweet little brown plastic serving dishes in a variety of shapes, a brown plastic tray and the opportunity to sit with beautiful people. But before I could get too over-excited I was roundly told off: 'Ma'am, you must be keeping dishes on tray; bringing food to dishes, not bringing dishes to food – much dirty splashing is happening. And no double-dipping.'

This last comment was addressed to a large, bearded American who had reached across me to dip his personal spoon and white robe in the Bhopali Mixed Vegetables. He wasn't the only one. In fact, there was a lot of elbowing and impatience going on amongst the serving dishes – it was everyone for his own chapatti. I tried to find this behaviour a reassuring sign that I was on planet earth amongst real people, despite most appearances to the contrary, but actually I just got pissed off – how rude.

Only a few people were in civvies. The candlelit courtyard contained at least three hundred white robes and, inside this uniformity, every nationality under the sun – especially Japanese people. Pramsu, a square-faced native of Tokyo, introduced himself.

'I like your name – but isn't it unusual for a Japanese person?' I asked.

Pramsu laughed, his gold-rimmed glasses glinting in the candlelight. 'Oh no, Lucy, this is not my birth name, this is my *sannyasin* name. I gave my photo and birth date and they gave me my name.'

'Who is "they"?'

He shrugged. 'Mysterious people in a small hut somewhere here. I like the name – it means "scholar",' he said proudly.

'Yes, it suits you,' I agreed. Pramsu bore a startling resemblance to an owl. 'What does "*sannyasin*" mean?'

Pramsu adjusted his glasses and blinked. 'It usually means renouncement of the world but for Osho it means renouncement of the old way. The new name signifies a new life – a new start. If you stay here two weeks you can get a *sannyasin* name, too. This place is a Buddhafield – an energy field for newborn people to meet fellow Buddhas. It's a very nice place.' He smiled happily.

'Ah, but I can't enter the Buddhafield until tomorrow when I have had my HIV test,' I replied.

Pramsu fiddled with his glasses again. 'You are here now so be here now,' he said wisely. 'Osho says – if you live only in the future you get stuck with your ego. If you live here, in the now, the ego disappears.'

'What else did Osho say?' The Swoony Swami would have been

cross with me – I'd been neglecting my *svadhyaya niyama*. I hadn't done as much spiritual homework as I would have liked, what with all the hugs, houseboats and nativity plays.

'Actually, Osho had no philosophy, no rules – he took from all belief systems and religions, from Buddha, Jesus and Krishna to Lao Tzu and Zorba the Greek.'

'A sort of spiritual pot pourri?'

He looked confused but ploughed on. 'He told his *sannyasins* not to believe anything until they'd tried it themselves – not to follow one system, not to depend on anyone.'

It was my turn to get confused. 'I thought he said that if you followed the *Raja* yoga path laid down by Patanjali you'd become enlightened – that it was a certainty.'

'Yes, he thought Patanjali was one of the greatest Indian thinkers of all time but he didn't say, "OK, now follow only Patanjali." He said enlightenment happens differently for everyone. The mistake of religion is that individuals impose their own experience on the whole of humanity.' Pramsu began to get quite heated. 'Why should everyone follow Christianity just because it worked for Jesus? Osho says find your own path to enlightenment. For one person it might be Dynamic Meditation, for another, dance, for another, music, for another, laughing. Anything that quiets the mind, helps you become what Osho called "no mind", is good.'

'So, I'm guessing no *asana* classes?' I said, disappointed. I had assumed that because Osho was a big fan of Patanjali there would be lots.

'No, *asana* practice takes too long – we just don't have days, or even hours, to spare any more, and it's too controlling, too systemized. Osho believed you need cathartic meditation techniques to quiet the Western mind but—'

The large American man with the Bhopali Mixed Vegetables on his white robe interrupted. 'Sweetheart, there are plenty of ways to get physical here beside yoga,' he breathed heavily, 'if you're interested.'

I didn't think, on balance, that I was.

The man in maroon was flirting with the girl in maroon. Actually, this was an observation I would make every minute of every hour of every day during my stay here, but my first recording of it came at the Visitors Centre when I checked in for my HIV test.

'You look great,' said the man in maroon in front of the HIV test check-in desk.

'Thank you,' said the blonde sex goddess in maroon behind the HIV test check-in desk.

'I'm so glad to see you're back. I hope we can connect later for a coffee,' said the man in maroon hopefully.

She smiled in a manner that suggested it was the third offer she'd had to 'connect' that morning. It was 9.06 a.m.

After the HIV test, it was 'choose a maroon robe' time. I hadn't had the test results yet – they would be given out at the end of the morning with our passes – so I was feeling a little uneasy. I was even uneasier when I saw the selection of robes on loan – shapeless, shapeless or shapeless. I came out of the changing room looking less like the come-hither sex goddess on the check-in desk, and rather more like a Harry Potter apprentice wizard.

The welcome tour began outside the Visitors Centre at the western gate, across the road from the black pyramid and the guesthouse. 'Follow me,' said the Italian guide, waving a large bottle of mineral water above his head. The crowds closed in and that was the last I saw of him.

The Water Bottle took us first of all to meet the cappuccino machine at the Plaza Café, which it claimed to have personally imported from Italy. Many beautiful people in maroon sat chatting and sipping deli-cious-looking cappuccinos amongst the foliage. As we followed the Water Bottle, it explained that the site had grown from 6 acres when it was originally purchased in 1974 to more than 40 acres, and had been responsible for the regeneration of the whole of this northern suburb of Pune. I don't think many people were listening – some couldn't understand what was being said and had started talking amongst themselves, and everyone else seemed too preoccupied with checking each other out. There weren't many backpackers, everyone looked pretty well-heeled, but there were three very hot Israeli guys who commanded most of the attention. Unfortunately, there were also two very hot Israeli girls so that put a lot of pressure on the remaining available Israeli man. He seemed to be handling it. Sadly my robe was rendering me, in true Harry Potter style, invisible.

The Water Bottle showed us a bewildering array of courses on the noticeboards at the Multiversity, to the right of the Plaza Café. Perhaps we would like to take 'Mystic Rose', which Osho created just days before he left his body. The first week would be spent laughing for three hours a day, the second week we would cry for three hours every day and the third week would be spent in three daily hours of silent meditation. The course was advertised as 'the most essential and fundamental meditation' and 'the first major breakthrough since *Vipassana* twenty-five centuries ago'. It was to prove a major draw – not surprising with advertising claims like that. There was a course already underway. Over the next week I would meet many people, mainly women, with puffy eyes and new best friends. They would sit together at meal-times – holding hands and staring searchingly into each other's eyes, breaking off occasionally to push Bhopali Mixed Vegetables around their plate.

Whichever course we chose, whatever our starting point, the noticeboards promised we would be able to leave the whole mess of our previous life behind and start a new one lived in joy and celebration. I wasn't sure about all of this. I was surprised that free-spirited Richard had spoken so highly of it – it was looking suspiciously like a cult to me.

The tour moved on. We visited the Buddha Grove where a group of white-haired, maroon-clad Beloveds were practising Zen archery, the first of 'Five Gateways to Zen', which would, according to the German girl walking next to me, 'enable them to experience the power of their *hara* – the location of their soul and their centre of awareness – as well as discover their vertical line'. We passed Beloveds hugging on the pristine walkways, Beloveds crying on each other's shoulders, Beloveds in designer sunglasses sitting on benches staring into space, Beloveds on the 'Zennis' courts – being told off by the umpire when they got too competitive, and Beloveds sunbathing in maroon swimming costumes at 'Club Meditation' – a leisure complex with an Olympic-sized land-scaped swimming pool, sauna and jacuzzi.

We were all mesmerized by the sight of so much perfection, and it wasn't just the beautiful maroon Beloveds. Like the guesthouse, every building looked as if it had sprung from the pages of the *Architectural Digest*, even the bookshop – a glossy, glassy fabrication with display tables and thoughtfully placed stools for browsing the thousands of Osho books, videos, audiotapes and Tarot cards. And in between every building nestled a bit of the orient – a jasmine vine here, a bamboo grove there, a Buddha everywhere. This was a five-star spiritual spa. Osho didn't believe in slumming it – he wanted his *sannyasins* to create a para-dise on earth. Why, he argued, should it be dirty and shabby when it could be clean and beautiful?

And then the Water Bottle led us to the Mirdad pyramids, a cluster of four buildings in one of the darker corners of the resort. It showed us into a room without windows, locked the door and hit us with the rule-book. First of all – how to conduct ourselves in the Osho Auditorium during the Brotherhood of the White Robes meetings; no sneezing, coughing, farting or burping. If you felt you were the kind of person who might want to do any of these things then you should take yourself off to the Omar Khayyam where you could cough and sneeze alongside others with the same nasty habits. If you had chosen to be in the main auditorium and didn't manage to control these mostly involuntary functions you would be summarily thrown out. And there would be no use trying to stifle a cough should it occur – the pyramid structure and the vast marble floor amplified any sound to the power of a hundred.

I was confused. Surely coughs and sneezes, like laughing and sex, suspend all other thoughts and therefore encourage a state of the highly desirable 'no mind'. Surely Osho would have been terribly supportive? Ah well. No time to ask questions. The Water Bottle was on to the next rule – no wandering about during the hours of the Brotherhood meeting. As I had found yesterday when I arrived, a strict curfew was imposed around the resort for the duration of the meeting. Neither would we be allowed in or out of the resort without our guest pass, which had to be renewed at a daily cost of 300 rupees (£3.75), unless we were Indian in which case it would cost less. (These domestic visitor tickets couldn't have been discounted enough – there were only a few Indians in the resort.) The pass could be paid for at the Visitors Centre using rupees but this was the only place real money could be used – apparently the rupee was a filthy thing and its circulation within the resort was forbidden, much like the HIV virus. Instead we should buy pink cards available in a variety of denominations at the Visitors Centre.

At the end of the session the Water Bottle unlocked the door and distributed our passes – receipt of which signified a clean bill of health. One girl didn't get hers. Everyone held their breath and pretended not to have noticed. After much embarrassed rustling of papers it turned out there had been a mess-up; there it was, at the back of the pack. Phew.

I had lunch at the Meera Café with Tamsin; she was staying in the Osho Guesthouse and we had smiled at each other in the state-of-the-art lift that morning. I had been very taken with her fine red clogs and very stripy socks. She had come looking for therapies that she could export back to her spa in the Caribbean.

'I tell you why counselling doesn't work,' she said. 'It's the counsellor's view of the world – you are just swapping one way of thinking for another. The cathartic confrontation therapies are the great joy of Osho, they really work. I'm taking "Mystic Rose" and "Family Constellation" home with me.'

Fifty-something Tamsin led a glamorous life. 'I had two weeks to spare after a meeting in London and I thought to myself, "Why spend it in that dreary place?" So I met up with some girlfriends in Goa, popped down to Kerala and now I am here for a week to look at these therapies.'

She leaned over conspiratorially. 'You do know Osho was a complete fraud, don't you?' she whispered.

I had to admit to having my suspicions.

She leaned in closer. 'I mean, he was a Professor of Philosophy, he was very widely read and he had a real talent for integrating the different spiritual approaches to enlightenment. Nonetheless, he was basically a confidence trickster who was only pretending to be a guru, and meanwhile amassed all those Rolex watches and Rolls-Royces that his rich devotees paid for. Isn't it deliciously ironic that none of his *sannyasins* have his sense of humour? They take themselves so seriously, it's hilarious.' She giggled like a naughty schoolgirl and pulled up the long stripy socks that had fallen to her tiny ankles. 'He definitely had the last laugh.'

Pronouncements made, Tamsin had to go – she had an appointment for a Psychic Massage and I had some shopping to do.

Being seen to spend money was not an issue at Osho's. Many of the Beloveds were wealthy professionals taking a break from law or architecture, and they didn't want to spend their money on dusty photos of their guru, or on tacky dolls and keyrings. Books, Tarot cards and courses soaked up some of their spare cash, but there seemed to be plenty left to spend on designer labels. A flash of Donna Karan on the inside of a cashmere shawl, a glimpse of Prada on a passing sandal and a sticking-out Calvin Klein label on a T-shirt worn under a robe were common sights here.

The maroon colour restriction was interpreted widely – apparently pink, purple, lavender and red were all the 'new maroon' – and, despite the sign in the changing room at the Visitor Centre proclaiming that 'a robe is a robe is a robe', robes could apparently be clingy, backless and involve criss-cross lacing. After an unsuccessful brush with a bottom-skimming T-shirt dress with matching leggings that I bought from an enterprising Indian woman's stall up the road and which resulted in too many cold stares from the Beloveds, I compromised with a more conservative 'old maroon' number from the on-site Meera boutique. It wasn't quite as curvy as the other girls' dresses, and had no lace trellis work, but at least I didn't look like Harry Potter any more.

Anyway, it was time to join the white Brotherhood in my other acquisition – a long, but satisfyingly clingy, white dress. Outside the black pyramid a crowd of my fellow Beloveds were gathering together to do some pre-emptive coughing. I hopped up the steps feeling quite pure, almost virginal, and left my new, 150-rupee, Japanese-style, white-velvet flip-flops – again purchased from the Indian lady up the road (I'd also bought maroon velvet) – with several hundred designer sandals in the stands provided.

The auditorium was as spectacular inside as outside, except that it was white. The marble floor stretched for acres. Projectors beamed blue and yellow images of prisms and stars across the high-pointed ceiling. The Brotherhood gathered; all wore shawls and many had bought collapsible chairs or fluffy mats. I found out why when I sat on the ground. It was f'ing freezing.

The band struck up and I went down to the front to dance and get as hot as possible before I had to sit down again. It was like a bad wedding party – the faintly Calypso beat gave anyone who was so inclined the excuse to make wave-like motions with their hands and arms. We had been instructed by the Water Bottle to 'allow the energy of celebration' to build inside us and not to waste that energy looking at everyone else. Nobody seemed to be following the suggestion. On the contrary, everyone was checking each other out. Several men, generally the larger ones, stood smiling appreciatively at the women's Calypso rhythms. Every so often the music would stop – a signal for the Brotherhood to shout 'Osho' and raise its hands in the air – all the better to dissolve into 'the ocean of experience' after which Osho was named. Following three final shouts of 'Osho', we had to return to our fleeces and chairs, or in my case, the marble floor. I had worked up quite a sweat during the Calypso beat so the ice didn't cut through while we were sitting in silence. My bottom only started to feel numb about half an hour into the video of Osho talking at one of his *darshan* sessions.

It was the first time I'd ever seen the man in action. It was a strange sight. I'd somehow imagined a 'Sex Guru' would be sexy – I'd read that he didn't have any shortage of admirers – that he gave special *darshans* to female disciples and had a long-term relationship with Ma Yoga Vivek (born Christine Woolf in Surrey), at least twenty years his junior. But Osho wasn't sexy – unless your sexual preference was for *Star Trek* characters. To me he was the perfect intergalactic hero, coming in peace and a flowing cream silk robe. The robe was a reflection of its time – the huge batwing sleeves and padded wing-tipped shoulders were the fashion of the eighties. The wing-tips were complemented by a cream silk, wing-backed chair in which he sat, his elbows on the arm rests, his immensely long and thin, manicured fingers placed thoughtfully in an open prayer position as his careful words of wisdom were beamed onto our screen, seemingly from a universe far, far away. His beard was long, grey and pointy, his hair hidden beneath a winter warmer hat. The only detail of his face that could be clearly seen was his remarkable pair of triangular eyebrows, the peaks of which sat about an inch above a huge pair of blacked-out Gucci goggles. Apparently the sunglasses were not worn for vanity but for sensitivity to light. Tamsin had told me that he claimed to have been poisoned by US government agents when he was in custody for alleged immigration violations in 1985, and that his health had suffered ever since. Other theories abounded – that the real cause of his ill-health was an addiction to nitrous oxide, administered by his personal dentist, or that he was dependent on Valium, or, rather more prosaically, that he suffered from chronic ME, asthma and diabetes. Whatever the real cause, in this film he looked ancient – much older than his mid-fifties – but timeless, as if he could have existed in any century. The only thing that dated him were the wing-tips.

He seemed to be speaking at great length about ashram politics – how women's jealousy had broken the first communes – but I could understand little. I found his pronunciation very hard to follow; there was a tendency to elongate the beginning of the word, flatten everything in the middle and taper off at the end – ancient became 'ainceeen', delicious was 'delleeseees'. But, although I understood little of the content, I found myself hypnotized by the slow rhythm of his phrasing. He claimed that he used words only in order to create silent gaps – that what was important was the silences between the words, and not the words themselves. This would help his audience to meditate; he argued that the mind wants to listen, and in waiting for something to follow, it too becomes silent. So much for the theory. I was just wondering if I was going to be able to follow the next bit of the sentence, or whether I would even know if he had moved on to a different sentence all together.

After the sociological discourse, the jokes. According to Osho even the jokes had a purpose – to keep us alert. Laughing was infinitely better than yawning. Their other purpose, like the gaps in his sentences, was to stop us from thinking. He said it's impossible to laugh and think at the same time, that when we laugh we enter into a deep state of meditation. Certainly the jokes were not difficult to work out – apparently he culled many of them from *Playboy*. I liked the one about the Martians and the astronauts best. Things were looking up. And then they looked down again.

Talking gibberish was supposed to help me break free of *chitta vritti*. I was interested to note that my gibberish moved firmly in the direction of China, veered off to collect some Russian drinking phrases and ate a few bowls of variously named spaghettis before returning home. But I have to say that, despite my superficial success, deep down I just kept thinking how stupid we must all look, sitting there talking complete nonsense, throwing our arms around and laughing hysterically. But I didn't feel I could abstain. The Water Bottle had told us that we must join in, 'otherwise you become the garbage can for everyone else'.

'Let Go' followed Gibberish. On the beat of a drum we had to fall down like a 'bag of rice' and lie completely relaxed on the floor. It was hard to feel relaxed on a freezing floor but there was worse to come. As we sat up, it became clear that men in white robes didn't wear pants, and that 'sack and crack' – a waxing technique made popular in London by girls who wanted their boyfriends to suffer the same levels of pain they endured in order to achieve the neat pubic landing strip of The Brazilian – had not reached Pune. I had turned a blind eye when I had seen the shadows of several liberated penises and balls enjoying the freedom of the Calypso beat, but here they were again, and now in hairy close-up. Should an underwear addendum be added to the rulebook?

I quite enjoyed the novelty of the Brotherhood meeting, but, as I sat in the Plaza Café and listened to the testimonials spilling from the lips of my fellow Beloveds, I felt that I might have tried harder to engage emotionally. I overheard one misty-eyed advocate saying, 'I never felt joy before I came here.' I needed to get with the programme. I wandered back over to the lists of courses on the walls of the Multiversity. Problem was, everything was so expensive. 'Mystic Rose' was £320 for three weeks and even the three-day courses were tipping £100. Osho readily confessed to being a guru for the rich, arguing that only they will know money can't buy happiness.

I'd already spent $1,000 on Mr V and another $1,000 was earmarked for the month-long course I'd be doing at the Krishnamacharya Yoga Mandiram in Chennai. I didn't really want to spend so much cash laughing and crying. The Cappuccino Gurus would roll up their sleeves and laugh or cry with me for the price of a cappuccino, although if I went on a bit I might have to fork out for a bottle of wine. But there was one course that I thought might be worth the money: '*Tantra* Energy'. There was an introduction at lunchtime the next day.

The Beloveds made their way up the stairs of the Omar Khayyam to a small dark room. A husky, sexy voice was sighing into the mike and gently suggesting we find a partner. 'Look into their eyes. Explore what is there,' she sighed. 'Feel your own sex.' She sighed again. 'Charge it and shoot the energy to your heart.' Another big sigh. 'Move around the room and make eye contact as you think about your sex. How do you feel?' Another big sigh.

Actually I felt acutely embarrassed.

'Now close your eyes and feel what you are touching as you brush slowly against each other. Slowly. No peeping.' Another big sigh.

I could feel hot breath and hot bodies, a mass of aroused dicks and keen, thrusting bosoms. I wasn't the only one peeping; how else would all the pretty girls and handsome boys have gathered in one corner?

'Get juicy. Mmmm,' she said, as if she had just eaten something delicious.

I had never felt more English.

'Now stop in front of someone and take their hands. Touch your sex to your heart energy. Soar together; you are joined in play.'

I stood before an intelligent-looking man who reminded me of my younger brother. I looked down. This would never do. Fortunately, we moved on quickly.

'Now close your eyes and find a new partner. Take their hands. Breathe together. Now open your eyes.'

I couldn't believe it. Hello, Barcelona! There before me stood a tall, muscular man with perfect teeth and olive skin. His moist brown eyes disappeared in a warm smile.

'Now tell your partner how your sex feels to you right now,' our instructress breathed.

'My sex feels open to you right now,' said the man I would later know as Miguel. His eyes disappeared again.

'And my sex feels open to you,' I said, blushing and looking at the floor.

'Now tell your partner how your heart is towards them right now,' she sighed.

'My heart is open to you right now,' he said.

I nodded, looking at the floor again.

'Cappuccino?' suggested Miguel.

Over Italy's finest, in the midst of the oriental foliage at the Plaza Café, we learned that we were completely incompatible. It only took five minutes.

Miguel was a numerologist. He took my birth dates and quickly worked out that I was a number two. Hmmm. 'It mean you are – 'ow you say – falling over a rock always.'

'Stumbling?'

'Yes, stumbling. But this rock, 'eet can teach you if you listen to it.'

'Listen to a rock?'

'The rock is telling you that 'eet is giving.'

'A rock that gives that I should listen to?'

'Yes, this year is a six year. It will be powerful for you. Two and eight are the most powerful numbers. I am an eight. But being powerful must be your intention and not your action.'

'Sorry, what do you mean?'

'Do not set out to act powerfully, only make it your intention to be powerful; then you are listening to your rock.'

I nodded, trying to look as if I had understood and was grateful. Fortunately he had to get to a meditation session so I didn't have to pretend for long.

The *Tantra* taster had left me with a lot of energy that the conversation with Miguel had done little to assuage. If I hurried I could catch the tail-end of the lunchtime disco in the Buddha Grove. The last time I had been there it had been full of the sound of silence as Zen archers drew their arrows in a state of no mind and experienced the power of their *hara*. This time the grove rocked to the sound of Madonna, Kylie and Cher. Two girls danced on a podium, allowing themselves to be 'possessed by dance'. One was Madonna on her *Like a Virgin* tour – complete with conical bosoms and suspenders; the other was equally spectacular in an iridescent blue net skirt with silver top, tights, platform boots and matching silver face.

Osho's babes were out in force, and they were all South American. I tried my best to imitate them but I was lacking some vital attributes – thick, wavy tresses that could be tossed in high-energy moments, cappuccino-coloured skin and a skimpy maroon number with lace trelliswork across its low-cut back. I watched transfixed as an arresting South American man with a noble nose and long black hair tied back in a strip of black leather, tangoed with a milky-white blonde. I'd never seen anyone tango to Cher before but by god they made it work.

As I watched the disco crowd letting go I began to wonder how much more they had to let go of. Everyone seemed to be pretty relaxed already. I really wanted to let go a bit more – the *Tantra* course might have helped but I felt the group thing wasn't my thing. It was a shame that I couldn't get past my uptight Englishness really – eighteen men had signed up, and only four women.

That evening there was a 'Celebrating *Sannyas*' event in the Osho auditorium. I sat with Rishi and Sargama at dinner. Sargama had just received her *sannyasin* name from the people in the little hut tucked away somewhere in the resort and now she was looking forward to her new life with Rishi, whom she had met here last year on a 'No Mind' course.

'Are you sure? It seems a big step,' I asked Sargama.

'I have wanted to go ahead with this for a long time – to work on my ego and conditionings, to feel truly free – but I always had so much doubt: what would I be leaving behind? And then I read that Osho said you should go ahead even if you have doubt in forty-nine per cent of your mind – otherwise you are denying your majority – the other fifty-one per cent. Plus I really wanted to show that I have surrendered totally to Osho and you can only really do that if you take *sannyas*.'

'Sargama is ready,' said Rishi, putting his arm around her and squeezing her tight. 'We have fallen in love with each other and with Osho. Osho said, "My *sannyasins* are pure love and I am pure love. It is a love affair".' His eyes misted up.

Sargama looked close to tears, too. 'I am really looking forward to leaving plain old Diane from Massachusetts behind, all those old fears and worries about not being good enough – I'm going to let them go this evening. Yes, sir.'

They squeezed hands and left for the auditorium.

It was actually a much more low-key ceremony than I'd been imagining – for some reason I had it in mind that they would be dipped in the still black pools of water that surrounded the auditorium and would arise coughing and spluttering and shouting, 'Hallelujah.' Something told me that it would probably involve hugging.

As it was, the band played, we waved our arms and then Osho spoke – a disembodied voice proclaiming in those famously broken sentences that '*sannyas* [pause] means [pause] freedom'. The crowd moved into a circle surrounding the five supplicants. Osho spoke more disembodied words, there was more music and then the crowd queued up to hug the shiny new *sannyasins* and garland them with flowers. Then they started hugging. Well, I'd got that bit right.

The next morning I hauled myself out of bed just in time for the 6 a.m. Dynamic Meditation in the Auditorium. The Water Bottle had rehearsed us in the art of this meditation behind the locked door of the pyramid. He didn't want us to make any mistakes when we came to do it for real with the rest of the Beloveds. It was one of Osho's preferred cathartic meditation techniques – ideal for those hard-to-break-down Western minds. We spent the first ten minutes breathing chaotically, and the next ten exploding – screaming, shouting, shaking and generally throwing ourselves around. I kept worrying about banging into my fellow Beloveds so I had to break the rules and peep every so often. The third stage was the worst – ten minutes of shouting 'hoo, hoo, hoo' as we jumped up and down on the spot, remembering to keep our feet flat to the floor. This killed my calf muscles and left me struggling for breath. I was exhausted. For the next fifteen minutes we just had to stand still, 'being a witness to everything that is happening'. Finally we spent fifteen minutes dancing – now that bit was fun. The rest I didn't want to make a habit of.

I went straight from Dynamic Meditation to *Samadhi* Silent Sitting. I suppose I thought that sitting still for an hour in front of Osho's shrine would be restful. It was certainly a beautiful place. The Lao Tzu building was surrounded by rock gardens and guarded by a champagne-coloured Rolls-Royce. Osho had owned ninety-three of them, making him the single biggest owner of the marque in the world. The aim had been to have one for every day of the year, but unfortunately he 'left his body' before this had been achieved. He made do with the ones he had – spending an hour a day driving up and down the private road his *sannyasins* had built him. The Rolls-Royce was, according to his *Autobiography of a Spiritually Incorrect Mystic*, by far the best form of transport for meditation and spiritual growth.

The car wasn't just used for meditation though. He claimed to have bought the first one for practical reasons – to persuade the banks that the commune was worth lending money to. The strategy had worked and the day after the purchase the company secretary had been offered money at the best rates, by every bank in town. The car was also a good public relations machine, leading to a big article in *The Times of India* – a newspaper that had never before printed a single word about him. And it may even have been responsible for some *sannyasin* recruitment – on the back of that article people came to see the car, and then stayed for the morning *darshan*.

I put on the white socks given to me by a Beloved so that I would-n't damage the marble floor with my bare feet and padded through Osho's well-stocked library, past his imported old-fashioned dentist's chair (his personal dentist and doctor were on call 24/7) into the *samadhi* shrine. The room was dazzlingly bright, with floor-to-ceiling windows, an enormous chandelier and many metres of pale-grey marble. I settled myself on a cushion in front of the shrine, underneath which his ashes were placed. I could feel his presence here; his eyes, in the picture above the shrine, appeared to be staring straight at me. There was a soft stillness in the air and I felt a sense of relief – but maybe that was just the relief of not having to shout 'hoo, hoo, hoo' and jump up and down on flat feet. It didn't last long. Thoughts of bananas and porridge were creating *chitta vritti* – I seemed to have built up a good appetite with all that jumping, and my stomach started to rumble. Loudly. The Beloved guard on the door came over and tapped me on the shoulder. I thought it best for everyone if I left before I was escorted off the premises.

I had a big breakfast with Michael the Belgian, and explained that fantasies about porridge and bananas had won the battle for control of my mind. 'Why battle?' he asked. 'If you try to control it your mind will win; you will strengthen its resolve. You must let it go. Observe it only.'

'Do you have much success with Dynamic Meditation?' I wondered.

'Yes, I go daily when I am here. At home I get up at four-thirty, maybe five, and drink a little hot water. Then I am meditating. Also before I go to bed I play the movie of my day, observing it only. Then I meditate again to calm my mind before I sleep. Do you "OM"? Repeat the OM *mantra* daily?'

'Erm, I haven't had much luck with *mantras*.'

'Perhaps you would allow me to demonstrate, Lucy. It might help you.' Michael pushed his chair back from the table and breathed in slowly and deeply. Then from the absolute core of his *hara* he let out a rich resonant 'aaaaauuu', which rose with his hands up past his chest and ended with an 'uummmmmm' at his third eye. He touched his hands to his forehead and bowed. There was a small pause. There seemed nothing for it but to clap.

'Awesome,' I said appreciatively. Truthfully I was beginning to find these conversations a bit of a strain, but I felt I had to give the place and its peculiar people my best shot. I wasn't going to get another chance to go on a trip like this for a long time, if ever, and I didn't want to dismiss anything without investigating it thoroughly – sometimes the most valuable things lie in unexpected places.

'You know,' said Michael, 'if you want to get some exercise,' I wondered where this was going, 'you could always try T'ai Chi. The master here is excellent.'

I went the next morning. I knew that my calf muscles wouldn't be able to cope with another Dynamic Meditation but I thought some gentle T'ai Chi moves would help ease me into the day. There was an early-morning chill in the Buddha Grove, and everyone was wearing at least three layers except our teacher – an authentic-looking, bald-headed man in a black robe. He took us through our paces; we Beloveds created a ball with our hands that we carried from right to left and moved up and down. I was beginning to flow with the waters of Zen until he told us, in a strong American accent, to 'keep your back straight, pull in your butt and use your abs'. Somehow this broke the spell.

I tried a couple more meditations that day – *Vipassana*, sitting quietly watching the breath for forty-five minutes – followed by a fifteen-minute slow walk, and discovered that neither that nor *Nadabrahma* Meditation – humming for half an hour followed by circular arm movements – were my thing. I was finding being in this place quite exhausting and needed some light relief. I was glad to see that there would be a disco in the Plaza that night.

The music was good and I danced on one of the platforms that lined the dance floor, mainly because it gave me a clear view of my fellow Beloveds in action. I had to do a double-take when I first saw Gorgeous George, and jumped down off the platform to get a closer look. Yes, he really did look just like his namesake George Clooney – but he had a very thick Italian accent through which I just made out an important opening line: 'You should have stayed on the platform, you dance good.'

I should have left it at that really; after all, he had suggested that I stay on the platform where conversation would have been impossible. But no, I insisted on taking things further. Turned out Gorgeous George had been travelling around the world for six years – India was his last stop before returning home to Rome.

'What work do you do in Italy?' I enquired.

'I in restaurant beezneez.'

'Oh, do you own a restaurant?'

Gorgeous George shook his head.

'Chef?'

Gorgeous George shook his head.

'I am waiter.'

I spent some time carefully outlining the workings of the restaurant business in London, and how long I had been travelling for, and exactly where I had been in India. Gorgeous George smiled and nodded and clearly didn't understand a word I said. There was nothing for it but to dance, so dance we did for the next three hours. I wouldn't say it was an entirely successful dancing meditation episode – I was too possessed by thoughts of Gorgeous George between my guesthouse sheets, scattering those fulsome cushions to the floor, to be possessed by the dance. Still, I felt that I was at least now moving towards the kind of meditation for which Osho was named the 'Sex Guru'. Imagine my disappointment then, when three hours after he first started throwing me around the dance floor Gorgeous George came to an abrupt stop. He said he needed to do some more courses before he would be ready.

You would think that he might have done enough – 'I am doing course works nine month. I try but it taking long time to clean me. No involve possible.' Who said anything about getting involved? He gave me a big hug and waved me goodbye. This was closely followed by a big hug from a round and hairy *sannyasin*, who had taken advantage of my still open but rapidly cooling arms and slid in for a quickie. 'Mmm, delicious,' he said, pressing himself against my hot and sweaty body. As Cartier would say, 'Eeuwww.'

The next day, I treated myself to lunch at 'Zorba the Buddha'. This upmarket gourmet restaurant next to the swimming pool was named after Osho's vision of the ideal man – one who enjoys 'the wholeness of being' – comfortable in both the spiritual and the material world. I sat on my own, overshadowed by the giant flowerpots, and tried to decide how to spend my afternoon. There was a choice – a film featuring Osho, a Sufi poetry reading and the ubiquitous meditations. Nothing was speaking to me.

A man and a woman took up residence beside me and, in time-honoured Beloved fashion, were soon discussing their relationships difficulties. The Billy Bob Thornton lookalike, his baseball hat worn the wrong way round, stared miserably into his Crêpe Pear Gorgonzola and Grilled Vegetable Salad and asked his pretty companion why the women he loved didn't love him: 'I vant to stop ziz and love but I cannot. Over and over I go. I am 'ere seven month – more and more course I do but no better getting.' He looked close to tears. The pretty companion smiled sympathetically and reached for his hand. The warmth of her touch unleashed a shudder of grief and out poured wave after wave of heavy sobs.

There was so much thought being given to how to live here – it was all so complicated, people were taking themselves so seriously. Suddenly I felt the need to get away. I polished off my Figs Praline and walked up the road to the Barista Coffee House – underneath the Sunderban, a 1930s hotel with sweeping staircases and gentle green lawns.

The Barista, part of a burgeoning chain of coffee shops, sold an array of Italian coffees, muffins and chocolate brownies, familiar to anyone who goes to Starbucks. Nothing Indian on the menu. I ordered a cappuccino and sat watching my fellow coffee-lovers. It was an interesting role reversal. There were several of my fellow Beloveds in the Barista, talking quietly and intently, self-important in their maroon one-pieces. The twenty-something Indian professionals in tight jeans and even tighter T-shirts chain-smoked and jabbered away to their friends, ostentatiously answering their high-tech mobiles at top volume, much to the irritation of the maroon-robed. I managed a chuckle at the irony of it all but the humour of the situation didn't make up for the sadness I felt at the disappearance of our cultural differences.

Sitting outside on the lawn, under the shade of a tree, I was joined by Miguel who had just done the first day of the 'Tantra Energy' workshop. I was glad to see him. Although we hadn't really, in the language of an Osho relationship workshop, 'connected', he was a handsome face on a pretty lawn on a hot day. Better yet Miguel had a friend in tow called Zack – a curly-haired native of Byron Bay, Australia. Zack spent his time healing washing machines with astrology, crystals and *Tantric* energy. He'd done a *Tantric* workshop in Mullumbimby just up the road from Byron and he was really pleased with the results – washing machines seemed to love it. Miguel had to go and meet Adriana, a South American girl he had met on the course, so he left Zack to show me the *Tantric* ropes. I was willing to give it a try. If it worked on washing machines …

'OK, Lucy, so we're going to whoosh our sexual energy up our spines, raise the *kundalini*, open our *chakras* and share in the bliss of *Tantra*. Ready?'

I nodded.

'Sit facing me with your hands in mine. Now shut your eyes, breathe deeply and allow *kundalini Shakti* to awaken. Feel the heat moving up your spine, opening each of your *chakras* – flowing up through *muladhara chakra* – the origin of your sexual urge. Did you know that every sexual urge in the universe is a cosmic act?'

I shook my head.

'Feel your body becoming lighter as your energy moves towards the dark blue of the *svadishthana chakra*. Breathe. Imagine *manipura chakra* is flooded with elemental fiery red. Can you feel the heat coursing through your body, Lucy?'

I smiled politely.

'Now open your heart to the vermilion lotus at *anahata chakra*, and let's flow towards the sixteen-petalled *vishuddha chakra* – the site of your soul, your *jiva*. Imagine the colour turquoise flooding the area with rich healing energy. Still with me?'

I nodded again.

'OK, so now all that vital energy is coursing towards your third eye – can you see the silvery white light of *ajna chakra*? From here we have a direct line to *isvara*, the Divine, the inner guru that lives in all our hearts, the best of ourselves. Let's move our desire up to *sahasra padma chakra* – feel the thousand petals of your crown *chakra* opening, merge with cosmic bliss, feel the love of the universe embracing you. Can you feel the charge pulsating through your entire body?'

There was nothing for it but to fake it. I breathed deeply, as if in the throes of passion. I imagined myself in Gorgeous George's arms. 'Yes, yes, yes,' I cried. I opened my eyes. Was that enough?

Yes. Zack was looking very pleased with himself. 'Babe,' he said dreamily, seemingly drinking me in, 'you look incredible. Your *ojas Shakti* is radiating out of every pore – you have an amazing glow, your eyes are shining, your cheeks are flushed.'

'My *ojas Shakti*?'

'Yes', said Zack reaching his arms around my neck in his excitement. 'Think of it, dude – all those hormones, all that sexual energy, coursing through your body, converted into pure spirit.'

I smiled again and thanked him politely.

He lit a cigarette and lay down under the tree. Pretty soon after that he was asleep. Then he started to snore.

Things were going from bad to worse. Men who wanted me to listen to my rock. Men who didn't want sex. Men who cried at the table whilst wearing their baseball hat the wrong way round. Men for whom I had to fake an already fake orgasm. Feeling distinctly moody and out of touch with the apparent radiance of my *ojas Shakti*, I left Zack to sleep and wandered back in the direction of the resort. Dusk was falling. There were scenes of relaxed perfection around every corner – a beautiful couple sat on a bench staring into the infinite black pools surrounding the Osho Auditorium, strangers hugged on the marble walkways, small groups taking a break from their therapy workshop sat on the grass and smiled through eyes exhausted by tears, a crowd lay on floor cushions amongst the fairy lights and watched a young dancer move her belly and ankle bells to the folksy rhythms of the *Bauls* – Hindu mystics from Bengal.

I went to sit on a bench overlooking the Buddha Grove. A middle-aged Indian woman with chipmunk cheeks came and sat down next to me. We smiled and said hello. I was pleased to see an Indian person; they were too rare a sight in the resort. I noticed that she had an Osho tattoo on her left wrist and asked her how she got it.

Ma Prem Satya had spent the best part of her adult life living in Osho's communes and raising two children. She had first been to one of his meditation camps in 1972, when he was known as Sri Bhagwan Rajneesh. She remembered him as a simple but charismatic man – appearing in a field in plain white robes and black slippers, and talking for hours to the assembled Indians. She'd gone to live in his first commune in Pune a couple of years later.

'They were good times,' she said. 'I used to dance and meditate all day. My children had several hundred parents. We didn't worry about anything.'

She noticed a big change when he returned from the USA where he had spent five years setting up a commune in Oregon, eventually getting deported for alleged immigration offences. He returned to Pune in 1987 as the Gucci-goggled guru.

'When he was alive it was all such fun,' Satya confided. 'Osho was a practical joker. The Rolls-Royces and the Rolex watches – we used to laugh about those a lot. They gained a lot of press attention and that was what Osho wanted. When he got the first few Rolls-Royces, the whole world started to take notice. There was always a journalist following him around, asking him questions and filming us. We used to enjoy all the attention and watching Osho play with these serious news men.'

'So why did you leave?' I asked.

'When Osho left his body, the young people took it over for sex and making money. I couldn't stay, though it broke my heart to go.' The chipmunk cheeks lost their roundness and Satya looked really sad.

I wished that I could have sat and listened to the black-slippered Osho talking in that field in 1972. Faking *Tantric* orgasms with an Australian who usually worked his wonders on washing machines seemed to be missing the point somehow. I realized that the thing locking me out of the maroon Buddhafield was myself. I didn't want to be here any more, in this personal development spa for wealthy Westerners spouting new age gobbledegook. Anyway, the endless therapies didn't seem to be working. Osho's followers might have been better looking and better fed than Amma's devotees but they seemed to me to be living in the same bottomless pit of neediness. I didn't want their hugs or their Figs Praline. I didn't want to drift along temperature-controlled marble walkways. I wanted to get back to the mess of India. It had only been a week but it felt like a lifetime.

The next morning I took a rickshaw into Pune. It didn't take long to leave behind the cool suburbs and manicured gardens of Koregaon

Park. I breathed deep. Ah, the sweet smell of pollution, the chaos of an Indian city, the unrelenting heat. Actually the city looked very cosmopolitan – there were Barista coffee shops everywhere, three HSBC banks and lots of young professionals driving brand-new cars, but it was still unmistakably India. Cars, rubbish and cows flowed around us, horns sounded incessantly. We sat in a traffic jam and my rickshaw driver hassled me to visit 'very good shop' for 'half-price fare'. I grinned from ear to ear. I couldn't have been happier.

The driver dropped me at the Ramamani Iyengar Memorial Yoga Institute in Shivaji Nagar, opened in 1975 and named in memory of Mr Iyengar's beloved wife. The building, like Mr Iyengar's body, was a temple to yoga. Shaped like a semicircular pyramid, it was constructed to echo Patanjali's eight-fold path of yoga, with eighty-eight steps and eight beams radiating towards eight external columns. Outside there were two idols of Patanjali; inside Iyengar himself was the prevailing, rather fierce-looking, force. His craggy features – a heavy-set brow, square jaw and clamped-shut mouth – dominated the entrance hall from a large oil painting, the glint in his eye as sharp as the light playing off the gold medallions on display around the room.

It felt good to be back in familiar territory. The reception contained only yoga students awaiting the arrival of Pandu Rao, the Institute Secretary. No maroon robes, no hugging and no beautiful people. Just earnest faces, robust bodies and sturdy legs in the school uniform of curiously old-fashioned pleated and cuffed baggy white shorts. The glass cabinets around the walls housed the memorabilia of a lifetime devoted to yoga.

Iyengar had taken it up in 1934 at the age of sixteen, a student of his brother-in-law, Sri Tirumalai Krishnamacharya, who was also the Mysore royal family's teacher. Krishnamacharya taught Iyengar, who had suffered malnutrition, malaria, typhoid and tuberculosis as a child, the basic *asana* practice that would improve his health. Sent to Pune by his guru in 1937, he survived early financial hardships and extreme physical challenges to become, as the brochure put it 'a legend in his own time', teaching yoga to Yehudi Menuhin, the Queen Mother of Belgium, the Indian cricket team and police force (including a special class for commandos), and the good people of Pune.

Pandu arrived and took up residence behind a desk in the entrance hall. He looked stern. I asked him whether I might be able to do some classes. The answer was a very firm no. The school's classes were hopelessly oversubscribed – foreign students had to secure their admission three years in advance and be registered with a qualified *Iyengar* teacher. I had done neither of these things. Pandu was polite but I could tell there was no room for negotiation. However, he did agree to show me the practice room on the first floor.

It looked like something out of the 1950s – a huge light space packed with people in white shorts and the props for which Iyengar was famous. Back in the forties Iyengar had used real bricks and metal road-rollers to help him ease into the more elusive *asana*. Nowadays the frightening array of ropes, pulleys and blocks were lovingly crafted specifically for their purpose.

And then, in an unexpected show of generosity, Pandu let me go down to the library. It was a very pleasant light room, although a little cramped with students and the thousands and thousands of books, which were carefully ordered behind glass and wood panels. Although it was well stocked it wouldn't have caused me quite the excitement that it did had it not contained the presence of Mr Iyengar himself. Pandu allowed me to go with a firm warning: 'Do NOT talk to Mr Iyengar.' I agreed readily; I had no idea what I would have said to this living yogic legend.

Mr Iyengar looked a little more portly and older than his oil painting, but much less fierce. He had the same bushy eyebrows, craggy features and thin, shoulder-length hair, but his eyes sparkled with the light of someone who has spent their life doing what they love; he smiled easily and laughed often. He was talking to a man about a forthcoming medical yoga book as he signed the certificates of the newly graduated. He exuded an air of great patience as this man, overcome with enthusiasm, gabbled away. The eighty-five-year-old Mr Iyengar smiled, nodded and chipped in, when he could, with the tireless enthusiasm of a man of twenty, betraying none of the health problems he had experienced as a child. I browsed the shelves, picking up books in Sanskrit and Hindi as I stole occasional glances at the great man, and the librarian watched me like a hawk. Joining five or six of his students at the long table that dominated the room, we pretended to study as we surreptitiously drank him in. His presence seemed to have a calming effect on us all. My *chitta vritti* began to slow right down and the only thing that gave rise to any continued whirlings was the awesome amount of jewellery on display. His white *kurta pyjamas* provided the perfect backdrop to a medallion, bracelet and several rings, all in gold.

I stayed as long as I felt Pandu's patience would allow. Smiling shyly at the Living Legend as I left, I received a really warm smile back. Perhaps I could get over my fear of those ropes and blocks. Perhaps I should find myself an *Iyengar* teacher when I returned to England and come back to Pune in three years' time. Perhaps.

I went to thank Pandu and met Sue from Edinburgh on the way out. I told her that I was disappointed not to be able to study at the institute now. She was sympathetic and suggested that I try one of Iyengar's senior disciples. There were lots up in Rishikesh apparently – the place where the Beatles and Greg's aunt had discovered the Maharishi Mahesh Yogi.

'Bramacharya Rudra Dev would be a good choice,' she said. 'He runs the Yoga Study Centre up there – apparently he has a rather militaristic style of teaching but he would be worth a look. And, come to think of it, the International Yoga Festival at the Parmarth Niketan ashram kicks off at the beginning of February. I don't know how much time you have, Lucy, but that would definitely give you plenty of choice.'

I went directly to the travel agent and bought a flight north, to Delhi, the closest big airport to Rishikesh, in the foothills of the Himalaya. I left the next day and was not sorry to see the back end of Osho's paradise. I returned to the dirt, noise and cows of India with joy in my heart.

~ 9 ~

'Stretch out upper eyelashes'

I woke in a state of high excitement. Here I was in Rishikesh – the self-styled 'yoga capital of the world'. My flight was supposed to arrive in Delhi in the morning, leaving me plenty of time to make the 220-kilometre journey north to Rishikesh. But a heavy fog had hung over the city for three days and all planes were delayed. I arrived late-afternoon to find the roads as congested as the skies. My Ambassador joined Delhi's rush hour in a slow, sad crawl past the slums on the outskirts of the city. I watched children picking though rubbish tips and small boys playing cricket with planks of wood as we sat bumper to bumper with shiny Hondas belonging to some of India's 300 million middle classes.

As we moved further north our travelling companions became brightly coloured lorries laden with sugar beet, milk churns, bullocks and farm workers. Darkness fell and a journey that had simply been slow became terrifying as my driver, Ekavir, decided that he wanted to make up for lost time and began to drive like a maniac. I had three near-death experiences that night, the last of which nearly resulted in an ignominious end – squashed between a cow and sugar beet wagon. By the time we got to Rishikesh, nearly eight hours after we had left Delhi, it was pitch-black outside and too late to haul my suitcase across the long footbridge over the Ganges to the Parmarth Niketan, the ashram that would be my home for the next three weeks. On Ekavir's recommendation I ended up at the Great Ganga (Indians call their holy river the Ganga), a large new hotel in Muni-ki-reti opposite the Parmarth Niketan. I'd stay for one night and go to the ashram in the morning.

Stepping on to my balcony the next day, I could just make out the pink clock tower of the Parmarth through the mists rising from the broad grey and silver slate of the slow-moving Ganges. I shivered in the damp morning air – I was more than two thousand kilometres from the nearest palm tree now. Much closer, and just visible in the mist, were the mountain ranges of the Garwhal Himalaya and the 'Char Dham' – the four hillside pilgrimage shrines from which the holy rivers begin their descent. Grey-haired monkeys with shining, boot-black faces came to join me, and a group of three sat on the balcony railing watching me eat my breakfast, their black, leather-glove hands moving in imitation of my own, their eyebrows raised.

More monkeys watched as I crossed the swaying 225-metre Ram Jhula suspension footbridge, towards Swargashram on the eastern bank, home of the Parmarth. The bridge was as much a trading centre as the streets that fed it; young girls and boys with watchful eyes and matted hair sold clockwork tin boats, coins, nuts and fish food – the monkeys dive-bombing any edible sales. The monkeys followed me over the bridge and took up their places alongside beggars chanting '*Hare* OM' and shaking their tins.

Swargashram means 'Heavenly Abode', but as soon as I had left the clean air circulating above the Ganges I was hit by a less than heavenly airborne mêlée of sharply acidic damp monkey fur, mangy dogs, cow dung, goat, old unwashed clothes, old unwashed people, dirt and dust, which overpowered the more cheerful smells of hot monkey nuts, frying popcorn, poppadoms, chapattis, samosas and dough balls.

I had imagined that Rishikesh, meaning 'city of sages', after its long tradition of visitors in pursuit of *samadhi*, would be governed by an ancient peacefulness. Not a bit of it. The competing CD shops created the most noise – Namaste's *'Jaya, Jaya, Shiva Shambo, Ma Devi Shambo'* did battle with Patala's *'Patanjalim, Patanjalim, Patanjalim'*, Ravi Shankar, Krishna Das and Mystic India. Second place was awarded to the wails of Minnie Mouse dancing on hot coals which emanated from the temples, third place to the white-robed American women clustering around the CD shops demanding 'the sacred chants of Devi and Shiva – for the folks back home' and wondering aloud, 'Y'all – what's the one that starts with "OM"?' In last place was the shopkeepers' endless patter: 'ma'am, very best price'; 'you look'; 'you buy'. Their shops contained a huge array of material designed to fast-track the purchaser to the spiritual world – carved icons of Krishna and Shiva competed for the spiritual seeker's purse alongside OM T-Shirts and a choice of sandalwood, basil wood or crystal *mala* beads.

The walkway was clogged by stray cows with painfully swollen stomachs full of paper and plastic, by more rows of watchful monkeys, by men pissing next to carts laden with cauliflowers and carrots, by bent blind women in widow's white, their cupped hands outstretched and their faces etched with suffering, and by some of Rishikesh's hundreds of wild-haired *sadhus* in their trademark orange robes. Some looked clean and fresh, others looked as if they hadn't had a bath since they'd hung out with George Harrison and Ringo Starr back in 1968. These orange-clad men were a familiar sight to me now, but for all that famil-iarity they hadn't lost their strangeness. To me they were still extraordinary – a reminder that the quest to live an eremitical life was still going strong in India. These men might be travelling up to the sacred shrines of the Char Dham by bus, they might have a Hotmail account, they might even have a bank account, but they still lived the ancient ideals as outlined by the Swoony Swami – they practised *bramacharya*, *tapas* and *santosha*, carrying nothing but a *kamandalu* or begging bowl, and stick. They were an inspiring, if slightly scary, sight.

It had begun to rain as I made my slow way through the din, but nothing could dampen the spirits of the Parmarth Niketan. There it stood before me, gaudily reminding me of Happy Mount Park, Morecambe Bay, where I had spent many childhood summers: metre-high, plaster-cast bunnies clutched blue rubbish bins; bright green benches lined pink-tinged, crazy-paving walkways; families sat under umbrellas in the rain. The only difference was that here the plaster statues depicted 'Meera in Divine love with Krishna' whereas at Happy Mount Park the gaudy plaster had been moulded into castles and windmills on the crazy golf course.

I followed some of the white-clad Americans I'd seen buying CDs into the ashram office. 'Hello, I'm Lucy. I'm here for the yoga festival. I rang and booked a room but I couldn't get here last night. I'm really sorry.'

'*Hare* OM,' said the quietly spoken man on reception. 'I'm sorry, too. There must be mistake making.'

'But I sent an email confirming my reservation.' I started looking for a copy of it in my bag.

'Yes, we are still having room, but yoga festival is March, not February.'

'What?' I refrained from shouting, I think.

'Madam, please be sitting down.'

I sat down.

'Trouble is coming,' he said, looking at my face.

I couldn't believe it – I had travelled more than a thousand kilometres for this festival – and it wasn't even happening for another six weeks. I couldn't stay that long because I had to be in Chennai on 8 February for the Krishnamacharya Yoga Mandiram course. I suppose I should have checked when I'd rung to book the room – but I had just assumed that Sue from Edinburgh was right. Iyengar's students always had an air of certainty. The man on the desk kindly offered me an early lunch as a way of removing the trouble from my face. I ate with my fingers. I was so distracted that I didn't notice until I'd finished eating that the two Indian couples on a day visit to the ashram had been using knives and forks.

I went to see the bedroom. It may have had a view of the distant mountains but it was freezing and untouched by a cleaner's hand – there was one helluva lot of hair in the plughole. They were charging $30 a night for this. My room at the Ganga, with its fully adjustable heater, hot water, clean bathroom, balcony and comfy bed would only be a third of that, if I stayed for a minimum of two weeks. But there was no room for negotiation here.

'This is best room. You don't like, you go,' said a different man on the desk, picking his nose.

So I went.

Where to?

Greg's aunt and the Maharishi Mahesh Yogi's ashram sprang to mind. I asked one of the white-clad Americans where it was. She directed me to follow the banks of the river for a kilometre. Off I set, in the rain and with no coat. It was becoming clear that it wasn't my day. There were the turreted ashram gates but they were completely over-grown with weeds and grasses. I decided to shelter from the rain in one of a hundred curious pebbledashed circular huts. Unfortunately, I chose a hut that already had an occupant – but Jo was very sweet about me disturbing her Transcendental Meditation. She told me I could learn it in England, although it would be expensive – 'They have to charge a lot to make you take it seriously,' she told me. I found out later that it is one of the richest spiritual organizations in the world.

Jo offered to show me round and her enthusiasm for the place was infectious. We took it in turns to sit on the cross marking the centre of the upstairs room in hut number nine, where, Jo told me, one of the Beatles had definitely meditated. Very soon we were back in 1968, imagining the band balancing their energies in the pairs of *yin-yang*-shaped huts with their sixties babes: Paul and Jane Asher; George and Pattie; Ringo and Maureen; John and Cynthia. We giggled as we imagined this famous band on their exotic quest for enlightenment, waking up surrounded by suburban pebbledashing.

Some of the huts still had great views of the Ganges but that was about all that remained of their sixties heyday. They had so many weeds forcing themselves between the stones that they looked like a collection of hairy coconuts. The huge hall that was used for meditation was still a dangerous place – not because impenetrable fields of energy were sending yogis flying across the room, but because there were shards of broken glass on the floor, and the roof looked as if it was about to cave in. Even the Maharishi's house was a ruin – all that remained of what would have been his throne was a bit of wood, which had now been put to good use as a step up to his terrace.

The rain had stopped so Jo and I sat for a few minutes taking in the clean air and the spectacular views towards the Hare Krishna temple across the now glassy Ganges. Jo told me that the ashram had closed down six years ago when the Maharishi had decamped to Holland, fed up with the ever-expanding Rishikesh encroaching on his peace and quiet. (I heard another rumour later, that the Forestry Commission had refused to renew the lease because of allegations of drug abuse at the ashram.) Whatever the truth, elephants were the only regular visitors now – walking through the ashram at dusk to drink from the river.

I was sorry to see it in such a state and a bit of me wanted to rush to the bank for a loan to turn it into Rishikesh's first boutique hotel. I could see the ads now – 'a soul spa for the world weary'. This seemed uncomfortably close to Osho's resort and made me feel slightly sick. On second thoughts – it was just perfect the way it was, even though it wasn't going to be sorting me out with a bed for the night, unless I wanted to become a *sadhu* and sleep beneath the stars. Something told me I wasn't quite ready for this.

I needed to find that bed so I thanked Transcendental Jo and made my way back over the swinging Ram Jhula bridge. I had no idea where I was heading so I was glad to see another familiar name – Sivananda. The Swoony Swami had told me that the Sivananda ashram in Rishikesh is owned by the Divine Life Society, a different organization from the Yoga Vedanta centres set up by Vishnu-devananda. Still, Vishnu-devananda had made it his base for ten years from 1947 when his guru, Swami Sivananda, the ashram's founder, had told him to stay. I guess I was hoping for another Swoony Swami but the buck-toothed *swami* wrapped up in an orange puffa, matching woolly hat and gloves bore no resemblance in looks or attitude. He told me there would be no yoga class for at least a month and that residence could only be obtained by writing in advance.

I was beginning to run out of energy but the sun was breaking through the clouds and I decided to explore a couple more options before I gave up for the day. Graham and Elizabeth, a couple I had met on that first Turkish yoga holiday, had been very impressed by Swami Veda Bharati, a disciple of Swami Rama of the Himalaya. Swami Veda Bharati was now a *Mahamandaleshwar* – a title that placed him in the top thirty swamis of India. Swami Rama's organization, the Himalayan Tradition of Yoga and Meditation, had two ashrams on the other side of town. Since Graham and Elizabeth had been sufficiently inspired by their trip respectively to give up their high-powered jobs in law and banking to teach yoga and run the Life Centre in Notting Hill, I thought it would be worth a try.

Swami Rama founded the first of the two ashrams, the Sadhana Mandir, in 1969. Another *swami*, also clad in an orange puffa jacket, gave *darshan* in its peaceful, flower-filled gardens on the banks of the Ganges. This was not Swami Veda – he turned out to be away in California until the beginning of February on a 'hide to write' break.

A tiny, shy Indian girl showed me a bedroom. I was feeling positive, even though it was $20 a night, until I saw the tail end of a rat disappearing through a hole in the wall.

Its sister ashram, Swami Rama Sadhaka Grama, had no rats but no personality either. It was like a retirement village – thirty-six modern, brick-built bungalows with neatly tended lawns and the odd old age pensioner sitting outside reading in the uncertain sunshine. If Swami Veda, the star attraction, had been around I would have been prepared to pay $35 a night but as it was it didn't seem worth the money, and I thought that I would feel isolated here on the outskirts of town.

I went back to the Great Ganga with the distinct feeling that I had come to Rishikesh at the wrong time of year. Lavenya, the hotel's long-haired and sphinx-eyed spa manager, took pity on me. A personal yoga lesson would be just the thing and she had just the man. 'He is great teacher. He is fantastic,' she said. 'I am *pitta* and am never calming down but he is having magnetic hands. He has been in *Elle* and *Marie Claire*. He is getting famous, especially in London. He is going to be famous around the world.'

An hour later I was in the magnetic hands of the handsome, dark-skinned, white-toothed Vinay P. Menon. Vinay turned out to be Lavenya's husband and a yoga teacher at the very glamorous Ananada five-star 'destination spa' in the mountains above Rishikesh. Lavenya showed me a copy of Zoë Williams's article for British *Elle* in which she had written about her pursuit of spiritual well-being at the Ananada. Lavenya used to work at the Ananada – which is where she met Vinay. There she was, pictured giving Zoë a lesson in her own trademarked fusion of Indian dance and yoga – *Niramayayoga* – and there was Vinay, elegant in starched white *kurta* pyjamas, teaching her *asanas* in an eight-columned white music pavilion with a gold-leaf frescoed ceiling, surrounded by neatly groomed lawns.

Vinay had a big smile and a passion for his subject; as the slow postures deepened he would push me gently, encouraging me to explore my limits: 'Feel it deep. Deeper. Feel it in your whole body'; 'Whatever is happen in your body let it come'; 'Breathe.' He worked very closely with me – alternately pushing, massaging and stroking my muscles into a state of peaceful surrender. By the end of the hour I felt as if all the tensions of the day, and several before it, had been coaxed out of me.

He gave his diagnosis: 'You are *vata*. This is why you cannot meditate. It is your mind always fluctuating – you are like the wind. You cannot stop it. It is not your fault. You must meditate only at the end of yoga practice – when you are tired your mind will stop. DO NOT try at any other time, it is not possible. Now, join me in chanting OM. Lie down, relac completely, your foot is relac, your shin is relac ...' And so we progressed through the body, until everything was 'relac'. 'Your mind is peace, your body is peace. You are the Eternal Self. You are Divine energy. You are consciousness, bliss absolute.'

And for the first time since I had been in India I believed that indeed it might be so. This was what I had been looking for – someone who instinctively understood me, someone gentle who didn't impose his own system on me, or his idea of perfection, someone who was prepared to work with what he found, someone who believed in me and possibility, helping me peel back the layers of that onion, revealing my purpose in life, my place in the world.

It was a bitter blow when I found out the next day that my experience of bliss absolute was to be short-lived – the Ananada were not happy with Vinay P. Menon's extra-curricular activities. I would have to find another teacher.

Mr Brajesh was an earnest man in a beige anorak, neatly groomed moustache and a slicked-down side parting. He also had immensely high buttocks. I met him by chance in the reception of the Great Ganga – he was a disciple of Rudra Dev, the owner of the Yoga Study Centre that Sue from Edinburgh had told me about. It turned out that Mr Dev, like pretty much everyone else in Rishikesh, was away until the second week in February. In compensation Mr B kindly agreed to take me down to the school himself. We travelled through the centre of Rishikesh town, banging our heads on the roof of the *tempo*, a larger shared rick-shaw, as we bounced over endless potholes, passing endless motor mechanic stalls where young boys worked hard refitting tyres to worn-out mopeds as worn-out men looked on from the sidelines, shouting occasional instructions but preferring to concentrate on smoking *beedis* and staring into space. Here, away from the spiritual seeker's stores, were the businesses that made the wheels of local life turn – banks, market stalls, electrical stores, biscuit and Bombay mix shops.

We turned down a small side street into a quieter residential area. The small school sat behind iron gates in a peaceful spot backing onto the Ganges. Mr B showed me the ropes, of which there were many. Twenty-four of them belied the cheerful red 'welcome' sign on the wall behind them. White lines marked out the correct placement of yoga mats on the concrete floor. It was still freezing at ten in the morning. I shivered. Those familiar *Iyengar* props – blocks, bolsters and chairs – were stacked away in a corner, but even from this safe vantage point there was something about them that scared the shit out of me.

We used the ropes to warm up. Mr B, still in his anorak, demon-strated. He hung on to one in each hand, his arms as straight as a broom handle, and dived powerfully forward on the inhale, exhaling as he folded into a standing forward bend. He repeated this ten times in ten seconds.

'We practise according to the season. In cold weather we must be vigorous,' he said. I must have looked doubtful. 'Come on. Do it!' He stood like an army colonel. 'Five times, come on, do it.' This was followed by squat thrusts. 'Inhale! Exhale! With force. Come on, Lucy. What is happening? Only ten? Come on, fifteen minimum!' This was yoga boot camp.

Then it was time for handstands. Again Mr B demonstrated, bend-ing his elbows three times as he lowered his head to the floor and back up again. He had to swing me into an upside-down position, and when I tried bending my elbows, everything else bent too and my head thudded to the ground. Ouch. I was relieved when he got out a folding chair – I thought we might have a rest – but no, I had to slot myself through the middle of it, lie on my back and rest my head and feet on the floor. I was finished off by the insertion of a wooden block under my sacrum and the instruction to 'relac'.

I would have liked to go back to my room to lie down but Mr B had other plans. He had appointed himself my unofficial guide and kindly organized a car to take me to see Vasishta Guha – a cave 20 kilometres out of Rishikesh on the way to Badrinath and Kedarnarth, two of the holy Hindu shrines that make up the Char Dham.

The road snaked high above the white sand banks of the Ganges. Here the river moved a little faster and the hills, thick with temples, acacia trees and palms, looked soft in the hazy sunshine. Mr B explained the legend of the cave as we made the steep descent to the riverbank. Vasishta, a sage, was one of the first creations of Lord Brahma. When his hundred sons were killed by the black magic of a rival sage he was so grief-stricken he decided to take his own life by jumping in the Ganges. But the River Goddess didn't want the death of such a holy sage on her hands so she carried him to the safety of his wife Arundhati, who decided to take him on a pilgrimage to help him forget the memory of his sons. On the way they stopped at this cave and stayed quite a while, several hundred years, in fact, whilst he performed *tapas*, before they moved on to southern India.

The present proprietor of the cave was Sri Chaitanyanandji. He was sitting on a low wooden table by the banks of the Ganges eating his lunch when we arrived. He was clad in an orange blanket and woolly hat, and giving poppadoms and *darshan* to the three respectful Indian ladies seated before him. He peered at me through his thick glasses, offering me a bit of poppadom, and a warm '*Hare* OM'. We sat with him for a few minutes and then went to explore the white-washed cave, the outside of which was decorated in pink, green and gold streamers and a frilly orange canopy. A big colour photograph of Gurudev Swami Purushottamanandji Maharaj, who found the cave by chance in 1928 when he was wandering through the forest, was on proud display on the dais, garlanded with flowers. He had actually lived in it for more than twenty-five years until a room was built for him nearby.

Entering the cave, the first thing I saw was a round pillar-like stone in a standing dish. It looked, to put it politely, like a representation of male and female sexual organs but turned out, according to my guide book, to be a *Shiva linga* – a *yin-yang* symbol portraying the eternal embrace of cosmic masculine and feminine higher forces. We moved to the back of the cave where Mr B pointed out a small gap in the wall. Beyond this, apparently, was another cave that went on for miles up into the Himalaya. In this cave were reputed to live a number of *siddhis*, beings with supernatural powers, doing *tapas* in their subtle bodies, not visible to the naked eye. Actually there wasn't much in this cave that was visible to the naked eye. It was very, very dark. We sat in the inner chamber and watched the candles flickering. I had been hoping that Gurudev Swami Purushottamanandji Maharaj, who had been dead since 1961, might appear before me as he had to several other Westerners. He had shown himself to a young Dutch woman, laughed like a child and told her that he was not an illusion but when she told him she wanted *gyan* or spiritual knowledge, he'd laughed again, this time wildly, and disappeared. No dice for me either.

After a while I got fed up of the dark and went to sit on a rock by the Ganges. Mr B followed and displayed a previously unseen sense of humour by standing on one leg in tree pose. Perhaps he wasn't joking. He clambered onto my rock, and we sat watching the white sand and afternoon sun combine to turn the river a brilliant sparkling turquoise. I breathed deeply and smiled. It was almost warm enough to sunbathe but something told me it would not be appropriate to strip off. We stayed here for an hour, just breathing the pure air, feeling the sun on our faces and watching the villagers work the fields of grain high above us.

At Mr B's suggestion I finished the day back at the Parmarth Niketan for the nightly *Arati* Prayers held on the *ghats*, or steps, overlooking the Ganges. Although we had got off to a rocky start – yoga boot camp really wasn't my thing – I'd warmed to Mr B over the course of the day and I really did wish him well, especially in his search for a wife. He seemed to think it would be pretty straightforward and told me: 'I am waiting to see beautiful girl and then I will say to my parents, "This one, please."'

At the ashram, young boys, anointed with *kumkum* and wrapped in regulation orange blankets, sat in three rows of three and chanted *Vedic* hymns, amplified by several strategically placed loudspeakers and a backing band of *tabla* players. They made a pretty picture, glowing orange against the backdrop of the fading light on a grey Ganges. A lifesized statue of Shiva sitting on a lion-skin over a pile of rocks, separated from the *ghats* by a few metres of water, cast a luminous though slightly eerie blue glow over the proceedings.

The two *swamis*, young moustached men with slicked hair and razor-sharp partings, led the crowd through the ceremony – lighting a big fire which burnt in a red, white and blue bunker, choosing a lucky few to come down to the fire for prayers and then taking the *Arati* lamp into the crowd to be waved in the shape of an OM. This was not without its difficulties as the lamp, much bigger than that used at the Sivananda Ashram in Kerala, bore a marked resemblance to a heavy copper saucepan that was on fire. Some of the older impeccably groomed Indian ladies, dressed in emerald-green saris with heavily embroidered borders, really struggled to hold onto it, and disaster was averted only by the intervention of an eldest son with strong arms.

I realized as I watched that I'd been expecting the Indian people to be proficient in all forms of worship, spirituality being something of a national industry, but these Delhi urbanites on a three-day mini-break to the pilgrimage sights of the Char Dham were no more familiar with these ancient ceremonies than the Westerners in the crowd. Actually the Westerners resident in the ashram were much more familiar with them than the Delhi weekenders. It was strange to think of these long-term residents, disenchanted refugees from Atlanta and New York, knowing more about the *Vedas* than the good people of Delhi, whose city was fast-tracking its way to modernization. Us visitors struggled on together, the *swamis* bearing it all with looks of great concentration.

I spent the next couple of days trying, in the pouring rain, to find an ashram, a teacher or both. I couldn't understand why it was proving so hard – this was supposed to be, after all, the 'yoga capital of the world'. The walls were plastered with the remains of ads for spiritual experiences of every kind – hungry goats and cows had eaten many of these experiences, and were presumably now reaping the benefits – but there was enough paper remaining to see that there were yoga classes at the Green Hotel and the Yoga Hut, meditation classes everywhere, astrology, 'speak Hindi in ten days', and even palmistry – 'Learn art of hand reading in just seven days. First time in Holy City, in a lucid style'.

I tried Yoga Niketan – an ashram that had once been featured on Japanese telly and had since become a home from home for trainee yoga teachers from Tokyo. The classes, held in a warm hall on a red carpet – two attributes worth signing up for in themselves – were gentle and flowing. The ashram was situated at the top of some very steep stone steps; this elevated position gave it great views out across the Ganges towards the mountains, and blocked out all the noise from the busy road below. The only problem was you had to stay in the ashram for a minimum of fifteen days to be able to attend the classes regularly, and you had to sign a form saying you would 'solemnly abide' by the ashram's thirty-one rules. The usual prohibitions against alcohol, meat, onion and garlic were joined by compulsory attendance at all meditation and *asana* classes and a 9.30 p.m. lock-in. I asked to see a room – no sign of rats but it was dark and damp.

Nonetheless, I might have been persuaded except that everyone looked so ill. The yoga class I had attended had been interrupted by a few hacking coughs and several of the students' faces bore the pale glow of fever. I was also a bit worried by the sight of several mattresses drying in the sun, giving the playful monkeys a trampoline fun park. No thanks, not even for 200 rupees a night, including all meals and classes. I flagged down a *tempo* and headed north in the company of some very serious schoolchildren up to Lakshman Jhula – the quieter end of Rishikesh – to see Primod at the Yoga Hut. We had a chat and he seemed perfect; he taught slow classes to small groups, but he was fully booked until February, of course.

I wandered down the steep path lined with orange-clad *sadhus*, in every size and shade of fade, chanting '*Hare* OM' and banging their begging bowls, and into a wide open market place in which a barefoot boy in an orange bobble hat and ancient dusty trousers was riding a bicycle wheel across a tightrope for rupees. I studied the crowd as they watched him. They were fairer than the southern Indians, their faces open, trusting. Some had been born in the town, or in nearby Haridwar; others were mountain people, who had travelled down through the alpine meadows, snow peaks and black ranges of the Garhwal Himalaya to Rishikesh, hoping to supplement the meagre living they made from their ten or eleven cattle, goats or sheep by selling the shawls, beaded purses and rabbit fur hats that they and their fellow villagers had made. They seemed more relaxed, more at peace with the world, more content with the simple life than the southerners I'd met. Uttaranchal, bordered by Tibet in the north-east and Nepal to the south-east, was quite remote, and Rishikesh, in the west of India's twenty-seventh state, felt old-fashioned, its tourism confined to yoga classes for which it charged too little, and the spiritual souvenir stalls. The town's character remained intact – there were no Barista coffee shops here, no shiny cars, very few mobile phones. The travellers I met mirrored the locals; getting here had required some effort, and once they had made it everyone wanted to relax. They would settle down, stay a while, enjoying the fresh air and (sometimes) blue skies, away from it all.

Continuing downhill towards the Ganges, I came to the pebble-floored Café Devraj, otherwise known as the German Bakery. The rain had made room for some sunshine and the view over the now green river towards the red-and-white turreted Rayambakeshwar Temple on the opposite bank and Lakshman Jhula, Ram Jhula's older but longer and equally swinging sister bridge, revived my slightly dampened spirits. There were always lots of chilled-out travellers here, gathered on the wooden benches to enjoy the views and exchange travel tips: Where was the best white water rafting? Who wanted to go trekking in the Garhwal looking for snow leopards? Did anyone want to share a ride to the Raj-era hill station Mussorie? Sipping my hot chocolate and savouring a chocolate nutty ball, I settled into a conversation with a Danish girl who wanted to organize some tiger-spotting in the Jim Corbett national park. We had moved onto debating the merits of a favourite traveller's haunt in Rishikesh, the Swiss Cottage hotel, so named for its far-reaching views of the snow-topped mountains when ... in walked Erik.

Taking me in his violet-velour-flared stride, he smiled and hugged me as if he had been expecting to see me, and ordered cheese on toast. Then he brought me up to date: 'After Sheshadri I tried *Ashtanga* with Sharath, Pattabhi's grandson, but it didn't suit me. I left Mysore shortly after you and came up here – it has taken me more than a month to settle in Rishikesh. I tried *Ashtanga* and *Iyengar* here also – but all these systems, they are not working for me. It's all too much about the body, I think about the body too much and I need to be elsewhere. Primod at the Yoga Hut – do you know him?' I nodded. 'He does meditation and *pranayama* and I like it very much. We are on a twenty-four-day cycle, the three of us. This, with my singing classes, opens up my chest and I am free.' Erik burst into a quick round of scales – 'doh, reh, me, fah ...'

– to demonstrate his new freedom, and stared dreamily out at the fast-flowing Ganges.

I explained that I would have liked to study with Primod but that he was fully booked. Who else did he recommend?

'I would go to Pankash at the Green Hotel – he trained with Rudra Dev but he has a sense of humour. You might like him. If you go, give my love to Kazu. Is that the time? I must go for my singing class.'

I didn't see Erik again; the ground between us seemed to have shifted. Perhaps Ben had been our glue.

I went to Pankash's class at five o'clock that same day. The Green Hotel was tucked round the back of the Parmarth Niketan, and the yoga room was tucked away at the back of the hotel, past a huge generator and up some very narrow iron stairs. The room contained a total of three fitted carpets, none of which fitted. There were twelve students waiting for Pankash, including Transcendental Jo and a long-haired, muscular Japanese man I took to be Kazu, who was watching himself perform a seated sideways bend in the mirror that ran the length of one of the walls.

Pankash's quiff bounced into the room several beats before the rest of his head. He was tall and slim with boyish good looks and a slightly quizzical expression. Transcendental Jo told me that he was now twenty-nine and had been practising since he was fourteen. He used to do seven hours of yoga a day but had scaled this back to two – which he did before he gave his first class at 8 a.m. His body certainly bore testimony to the power of yoga – it was long, lean, flexible and strong, the perfect teaching tool.

We began with a chant and then went straight into a round of sun salutations to get us warm – there had been a power cut and the room was freezing. He didn't seem to feel the cold, however, and walked around in nothing but a pair of small black nylon shorts and a gold medallion – perhaps in emulation of Mr Iyengar. The rest of us shivered in at least three layers.

After the sun salutations the class turned into a knees and hips workshop. It didn't take long for him to home in on me. Transcendental Jo told me afterwards that he did this to all of his new students but I didn't know that at the time and felt humiliated by his step-by-step deconstruction of my *virasana*, or 'hero's pose'. I thought I was looking rather good, quite heroic in fact. My back felt straight to me, and I was sitting between my legs with parallel thighbones and my bum firmly on the floor.

'Come. Come,' said Pankash. The students gathered round me. 'You see here. Look at the ankle and the foot – how they are out of place. Now place them by the body – tight in – come on!'

I thought that's what I'd been doing but I made an effort to comply with the regulations that were being shouted at top volume.

'Now roll the patella out and spread out the little toes. Where is the buttock?'

The buttock had lifted up as the little toes had spread out.

'What is happening to base intelligency?'

I wasn't sure that I knew what that was, let alone what was happening to it.

'Rotate the skin on your right thigh to the left and the skin on your left thigh to the right. Do it! Understand?'

I nodded in imitation of one who had.

'Hah!' he exclaimed.

We moved into a series of forward bends and back bends – motivated by a constant stream of exhortations: 'Yes, squeeze it, come on!'; 'Tight it. Tight it!'; 'Lift the inner groin. Lift it! Lift it!'; 'More down, more, more, isn't it!'; 'Squeeze it, squeeze it!'; 'Stretch out upper eyelashes!'; 'Stretch the wrinks, stretch it, stretch it!'

Most of my fellow students were physically strong and flexible – they had no problem stretching out their 'wrinks' (the wrinkles on the back of their knees) or their upper eyelashes. Kazu was the strongest and most flexible of all. The only thing getting in his way was his ponytail, and his desire to look in the mirror – which seemed to be in danger of causing him some neck strain.

After *virasana* came *adho mukha vrksasana*. To demonstrate this pose Pankash picked the luscious Lalita, a slightly podgy twenty-five-year-old Indian American with lustrous hair to her bottom, big black, kohl-rimmed eyes, pouty lips and an unreliable trouser zip.

'I don't do handstands,' protested Lalita.

'I know, so do it,' countered the masterful Pankash.

By the time she had been up in handstand for a few minutes the zip had worked its way back to its place of origin and was revealing some very sexy pink lace knickers. Pankash to the rescue. Slotting himself between Lalita and the wall, he put his hands around her waist, pivoted her back into an upright position and pulled up her zipper – all in one easy movement. The class blinked and moved seamlessly on.

Afterwards I went for dinner to Chotiwallah with Transcendental Jo and her friends. We were overtaken by the gloriously glamorous sight of Pankash and Lalita on his motorbike – their hair flowing in the wind. They could have been movie stars except that the sight of her pink G-string riding high above those unreliable trousers would have been airbrushed out.

Chotiwallah, meaning 'the fellow with the small tuft of hair', is a Rishikesh institution. Actually it's two Rishikesh institutions. Two brothers claimed their father had left it to each of them, and, in a Solomonesque ruling, the judge divided the restaurant in two. Now there were two elaborately made-up men with small tufts of hair gelled into rhino horns, sitting on thrones outside their respective restaurants. Competition between the two was said to keep the prices low and the standards of food and hygiene high.

Dinner was going swimmingly, the *thalis* were great and I was making some new best friends, until the moment I told them that I had just come from Osho's place and that he was a sex guru with ninety-three Rolls-Royces. No amount of protesting that it hadn't been my kind of thing either could have prevented the small conversational chasm from opening up. The party split into smaller groups. Transcendental Jo told me that Lalita was said to be a fan of the so-called '*Tantric* Romanian'. My friend Jim had met him in Rishikesh a few years before. Although Jim hadn't seen it with his own eyes, the rumour was that he held Miss Shakti contests in which wannabe goddesses tested their divine feminine powers by dancing naked around an oiled-up, elephant-headed Ganesh – apparently their sexuality was being used for the attainment of higher states of consciousness. Lalita would be leaving Rishikesh shortly to go and see him in his new home, Thailand.

The next morning's theme was 'walking like horses' and Pankash had us working in threes. Transcendental Jo stood against the wall in *virabhadrasana* II or 'warrior II' – one leg bent, one leg straight, both arms outstretched to 180 degrees. I pushed her bent knee and a fellow classmate assisted her inner groin so that it was flat to the wall. When she was released many minutes later she had to go for a walk around the room – she had indeed become a horse.

'See?' said Pankash. 'Normally you are walking from your legs, horses walk from their buttocks – that is why they are so strong. Understand?' We nodded. 'Hah.'

By the end of class Pankash had an entire stable of proud horses walking around the class. Kazu pulled out his ponytail and tossed his mane as he strode like a true thoroughbred in front of the mirror.

I walked back across the bridge like a pony on its way to the knacker's yard. Except that I was going to see an astrologist. The Colonel, a distinguished man with white hair and neatly trimmed moustache, had seen me browsing books on *Vedic* astrology in his shop and had suggested that I come round for a reading from his wife – an expert on the subject and a psychic. When she was a child, he told me, 'she would say what would happen and then it would happen – her family said she had a "black tongue". They did not like it – they were scientific.'

Mrs P and the Colonel lived in a modern pink block overlooking the Ganges, just up the road from the Great Ganga. She opened the door to their comfortable apartment holding her little fluffy dog, a twelve-year-old Yorkshire terrier called Tipsy, so named because as a baby he used to drink warm milk and keel over into a deep sleep. Something about the Colonel's demeanour made me resist the temptation to crack any jokes about whisky in the milk.

Mrs P fussed around me, her round body swathed in an expensive beige shawl. I was given very sweet *chai*, chowgri biscuits made of pure sugar cane and sesame seeds, and a plate of almonds, cashews and pistachios. I was beginning to understand why Indian ladies are often slightly larger than Western women. After the *chai* we did a brief *puja* – 'we ask the gods to help us make this reading accurate' – then Mrs P got down to business.

'Your seventh house of relationships is affected by Saturn – so you are having problems finding a partner. After seventeenth of February this year you will find. Do not search for him. He will find you. He is in yoga and spiritual things. He is not like you – he is older or not from your caste or not English. Late marriage. Love marriage. Good marriage.' What a relief. There then followed a warning. Mrs P looked at me sternly. 'You are worried someone will boss you but you must curb your tendency to stubbornness for a harmonious married life. You must reduce your fixed views.' What stubbornness?

'You are fond of arts and music and you love luxury. You are fond of society. You like pomp but you also turn from it ...Your motivation is spiritual liberation ...You will go from the professional to the spiritual ...You have a bold investigating nature. You will write a book about yoga, foreign travel is indicated here also.'

Writing a book was an appealing prospect, and I was beginning to really enjoy being in India; I could imagine selflessly dedicating myself to researching yoga centres around the world – Byron Bay, California, Bali. How about Golden Buddha Island in Thailand? Ulpotha, a yoga retreat in Sri Lanka? Purple Yoga Hawaii? Really, the possibilities were endless.

She interrupted my reverie, warning me that 'enemies are there but you will overcome them. With Taurus to help you the fruits of your labour will be realized. Fulfilment of one's earthly desires and artistic expression can blossom in this lunar mansion. There will be many books.'

The Colonel chipped in with a proviso: 'You must read a lot of yoga books and synthesize information for others. You must include the ailments that yoga can cure. Vishnu-devananda's book is very good. I have it in my shop. You will come.' I promised that I would.

Mrs P added to the shopping list. 'You must buy a yellow sapphire set in gold to promote wisdom and marriage. You must wear it on the index finger of your right hand on Thursdays. It must be three and a quarter carat minimum, ideally five and a quarter. First wear it on a rising moon fourteen days from today. Recite the *mantra* to Jupiter as you do a *puja* with a yellow flower and dip the ring into the Ganga.'

'Also, you need a coral ring set in silver for the ring finger of the right hand – wear this on Tuesdays for marriage. Do the same ceremony but with a red flower. You could also have a diamond ring for your marriage finger – the diamond is your birthstone. It is very important you buy your rings from a good store – you go to the gem shop by Lakshman Jhula. I'll give you a card. Very good stones. Very good results.'

The gem shop she recommended, nestling amongst the OM T-shirt shops and trinket stalls, looked at first an unlikely place to find a five-carat sapphire ring, but it turned out to have a secret inner chamber not visible from the street. I was asked to leave my shoes at the entrance and was buzzed through another door. The view took my breath away.

Brilliant white light danced off the refracted surfaces of hundreds of diamonds, yellow sapphires and rubies. Thousands of golden deities – Tara, Ganesh, Saraswati – lined the shelves. A porcelain Krishna played his flute, a full-sized head of a jade Buddha smiled a contented smile and there before me, smiling that self-same smile, was the round proprietor, Mr M. He sat behind a long counter containing more little lozenges of colour than the Woollies Pick 'n' Mix. Mr M offered me a cup of *chai* and wasted no time in getting down to business: 'This one is a five-carat yellow sapphire set in twenty-four-carat gold.' I put it on. 'You are wearing it on the wrong finger. For Jupiter it is your first finger.'

'But I don't like this finger,' I protested. 'See how it twists.'

Mr M looked at me sternly over his spectacles. 'When a doctor gives you medicine it is not tasting delicious but it is good for you. This stone is like that – it may not look good but it will do you good, bringing you marriage and prosperity.'

'How much is it?' I asked nervously.

'Twenty-nine thousand rupees. See, it is a perfect fit.'

'For two hundred and sixty quid it had better bring me a lot of prosperity.'

Mr M smiled patiently. I wondered idly if he was related to the Colonel.

The coral ring was much less.

'You see it is fitting most perfectly also. This is most unusual. These rings were made for your hands.'

There were so many beautiful gems in this shop – it seemed a pity to have to choose one over another. I asked whether he had one piece of jewellery that would channel the power of all nine planets.

'Actually we do,' said the ever-resourceful Mr M. 'Here is a Navratan bracelet – nine gem stones in gold settings. Thirty-nine thousand rupees. Each stone represents a planet.' He lovingly pointed out each stone to me – topaz, white sapphire, blue sapphire, diamond, pearl, catseye, coral, emerald and a ruby at the centre.

'That's a lot of money,' I said. 'They must only be bought as wedding presents or for twenty-first birthdays.'

'Oh no,' said Mr M, looking shocked. 'People are buying for themselves – like medicine. They must have one because it is good for them.'

He noticed me looking at a blue sapphire with diamonds from Sri Lanka. 'This one is good for *vishuddhi chakra* – for communication, and for marriage.'

'Mrs P said I should have coral and yellow sapphire though,' I pointed out.

'You must go with your instinct. This is the correct gem for you,' said Mr M firmly.

'Mrs P wont be upset?'

'No, her son is married to my daughter.'

And despite this piece of knowledge I somehow convinced myself to buy the diamond and sapphire ring. So much for *aparigraha*, possessing only what is necessary. On the other hand, a husband was necessary, so on balance it had to be a worthwhile investment.

I hurried back over the bridge as it began to rain, wondering how I was going to pay the airfare to Chennai when I'd just spent it on a ring, and got a *tempo* down to Ram Jhula. The road traced the path of the Ganges far below, now slate-grey and choppy. A *sadhu* stood underneath a tree, trying to protect his blanket from the rain, men clutched parcels to their chests, bracing themselves against the gathering wind, the postcard wallahs drew plastic sheeting over their stalls. I had been planning to have dinner in the company of one of the Chottiwallahs but the downpour led me to the steamed-up windows of the 'Eat Healthily Drink Pure Good Quality Less Profit' Madras Café. As soon as I walked in I knew that I wouldn't eat anywhere else as long as I stayed in Rishikesh. It wasn't that the décor was particularly inspiring – a stone floor and brown Formica tables – but there was something about the place that felt like home.

Perhaps it shouldn't have felt that way. The café's history abounded with dark rumours that the original owner, A. N. Manon of Kerala, was murdered by his wife's lover in a fit of jealous rage, or that he had been killed on a train, on his way back to Kerala, for the suitcase containing the season's profits. After this inauspicious start Mr Govinder Aggarwal of Rajasthan – a devotee of Sivananda and the Divine Life Society, had taken over the café in 1981. It was then that the café's reputation had been built in earnest. Mr Aggarwal kept the south Indian menu and it was the first restaurant in Rishikesh to offer *masala dosas* – crisp pancakes stuffed with potatoes, onions, turmeric and chillies – and extended the premises from a hole in the wall to its current ten tables. The café still bore several signs of an allegiance to the Divine Life Society – there was a large black-and-white photograph on the wall of Sivananda himself, beaming at the prospect of a large Madras Café meal. A Swami Chidananda wall calendar (the current president of the ashram) hung alongside a simple shrine, lit by a naked red lightbulb. The regular clientele were devotees escaping from the slightly-too-salty food served up at the ashram. These Divine Lifers were joined by travellers drawn by the promise, advertised on a board outside, of the highest hygiene standards. Together we sat, happily contained in that humid fug, protected from the roar of the generator, which kicked into action every time there was a power cut, by exotic walls covered in bamboo blinds, from which hung pink, yellow and green flashing fairy lights, a garish picture of Ganesh and a laminated map of the world.

Eating at the Madras Café felt like eating at a friend's kitchen table – the door would open and everyone would look up in anticipation of another smiling face. Conversations between the tables started easily, often facilitated by MP – the gentle-faced waiter with a blue sleeveless puffa jacket and kind eyes separated by a large amount of *kumkum*, a testimony to his daily *puja* to Ganesh, which he performed at home before his thirteen-hour day began. He was devoted to his wife, who was staying with him in his tiny flat in Rishikesh while she convalesced from an operation, and to his two children, who lived in a remote village in the Himalaya. Their grandparents were looking after them while he worked to earn the money for their food and schooling. He was also devoted to the fish held in a 2-metre tank – fishing them out with a net and restoring them only when he had cleaned the tank from top to bottom. There was room, too, in MP's big heart for his customers. He was as devoted to their happiness as he was to that of his fish, family and Ganesh, and seemed to have an instinctive knack of knowing what it was you needed before you knew it yourself. He seemed to me to be one of the happiest and most contented people I'd ever met – largely because he seemed to be able to find great pleasure in the small things in life. He had a lightness of being, a childlike quality that enabled him to find wonder in the ordinary, to be content on any street. I had seen this great gift in Mohan, Akshay and Taresh, the teenagers who piled into the rickshaw to help me find a room in Mysore. For me it had been a hot and desperate chore; for them an Elvis-enriched funfest.

Seeing that I needed warming up, MP took my green plastic mac and hung it up to dry by the washbasin. He gave me a towel to dry my hair and immediately brought me a hot ginger lemon drink. Over a plate of Himalayan Health Pilau, a Madras Café special, and *Paneer* Tikka Masala, I got chatting to the three Divine Lifers sitting at the next table.

Alan was a sign-painter from Birmingham who was finishing an acrylics and oil wall frieze depicting Sivananda's life in the *samadhi* shrine. It had taken him four years to complete and was a labour of love: 'I'm a painter, not an artist, but I just felt inspired to do it.' There was an American from North Carolina who wanted me to read him the phone directory 'with that Oxbridge accent of yours'. And then there was Mr Hospitality, a bald, ruddy-cheeked man with huge green eyes that were lit by devotion to his teacher, Swami Chidananda. He grew up in the Himalaya, fluent in Hindi, English and German, the child of journalists who worked for Swiss radio and newspapers. After he returned to Germany to finish his studies he worked for the Voice of Germany radio station where he was in charge of production for the English service. He'd been visiting the Divine Life Society ashram since 1953, when he was a young boy, and he'd recently made the decision to come and live in the ashram permanently. He'd just taken over the role of showing visitors around the ashram, and the holy sites in the Himalaya, from the general secretary of the Divine Life Society, Swami Vimalananda, the self-styled 'first servant of the ashram'.

I asked Mr Hospitality about the women in white robes that I kept seeing at the German Bakery. There were lots of them – all Americans, all with very short grey hair, similar to Amma's crew but healthier-looking. He explained that they were devotees of Shanti Mayi, an enlightened American woman. She was staying with her guru Sri Swami Hans Maharaji at Sacha Dam, an ashram he had founded in honour of his teacher Sacha Baba, who had lived, in time-honoured guru fashion, in a cave near Lakshman Jhula. We arranged to meet at the nearby German Bakery at lunchtime the next day and to go from there to her afternoon *satsang*.

~ 10 ~

'An ocean of love'

'I am love,' she said in a high-pitched monotone, the cigarette remaining clenched between her teeth as she spoke. 'What the world needs now is love. I would like to do away with all religions, churches, priests, vicars, prayers, chanting, any praising the Lord of any kind, and replace it all with love.' Plumes of Marlboro's finest smoke curled around a bob made grey by many years of such infusions. 'I am sitting here with you being love, you are also love. You must use your love to benefit others – cast it wide.' She motioned out beyond the confines of the German Bakery towards the Ganges and the mountains beyond.

Her audience, a young couple, nodded meekly. They had clearly given up trying to chisel an escape route into one of her sentences.

'In my hotel – I am in a hotel because ashrams are not love – there is love. The young boys that work there, and me – we are love together. A young Danish boy of twenty-three arrived, we met in the corridor and that was it – we spent the next three weeks together. He was like a son to me. Even though there is thirty years between us and I don't know how to access a website and he would rather buy a PlayStation game than a book – even despite these great generational differences, it is possible to create love. Then a Brazilian boy arrived – he was the same age as my "son" and now they are inseparable. I don't see them so much now but I remain love. I radiate love. Love is in the walls of this restaurant because I am here.' She paused to light another cigarette.

The couple, who had clearly been held captive for some time, took the opportunity to run away. They left in a flurry of dust and pebbles.

'Remember to spread your love,' called Marlboro Love after them, as she disappeared once more behind her smoke screen.

The couple turned up twenty minutes later, looking slightly ruffled, in the Sacha Dam *darshan* hall, on the banks of the Ganges. Its windows rattled in the howling wind, and monkeys played noisily on the tin roof. Hail stones rained down. The 200-strong crowd gathered and shivered beneath its white shawls. The majority of the devotees were like Amma's people – white, middle-aged women – but they looked happy and healthy; no international energy exchange programme at work here. One or two Indians stood curiously at the back of the room. Mr Hospitality and I sat at the back and waited.

ShantiMayi arrived looking as if she had just been to Sainsbury's. There was no golden jewellery, no crown and no throne. Terribly down-to-earth and no-nonsense, she sat on an ordinary, though large chair, her scrubbed, girlish good looks swathed in a regulation white shawl over a salmon-pink cardie. Pictures of her as a young woman, on sale in the foyer, revealed something of a Hillary Clinton makeover – a radiant honey-blonde with thin, gold-framed glasses and a high ponytail had replaced the plain brunette hiding behind thick lenses.

Initially I found it hard to take seriously this pretty white woman with the easy all-American smile. I was used to seeing enlightenment dished up in the form of wizened old Indian men muttering ancient Sanskrit texts in indecipherable accents, or younger Indian women doing the same. To be able to understand exactly what a guru was saying – and to listen to all-too-familiar discussions about self-acceptance, self-doubt and body image – was unsettling.

We got off to gentle start – a folksy guitar and *tabla* beat accompanied chanting led by an Eva Cassidy soundalike. Unlike Amma, ShantiMayi didn't flail her arms, or go into a deep hypnotic trance. Everyone clapped hands and swayed in time to the rhythm. But gradually, over the space of half an hour, the chanters' enthusiasm rose to fever pitch, and ShantiMayi punched the air with an ecstatic solo amplification of the chorus – '*Shiva shambo shankara*'. I found myself joining in – my flat pitch melting unheard into the crowd of angels. I wondered if her disciples actually had to pass an audition, or have voice coaching if they didn't measure up.

I had first noticed the ability of chanting to make me forget myself during the singing of the *Arati* Prayer at the Sivananda Ashram in Kerala. Millicent had told me that this was because chanting creates *mudita* or 'spiritual happiness'. She said that when she had chanted at the monastery in the Himalaya she had experienced feelings of boundless love, and had found joy in ordinary things – even in a bowl of watery soup. I had to admit that I'd been a little dismissive of Millicent's experience, but here the *mudita* was inescapable. ShantiMayi, remarking on her *sanga's* 'juice', said afterwards: 'Your voices were taking me way to the heavens.' I was surprised that Osho hadn't conceived a three hours a day chanting meditation as a process for getting to the state of 'no mind'. It seemed in many ways more obvious than sex or dancing, and could have been charged out at £300 a week, with the right teacher. ShantiMayi didn't charge anything for her voyages to the heavens – donation only.

The rest of the *satsang* was conducted like a chat between good friends – over the next three days I would witness many troubled devotees sobbing, explaining their problems and asking for guidance. ShantiMayi always listened intently and gave a response rooted in her 'love is the only resolution' philosophy, available on a T-shirt in several colours, alongside the books, tapes and photos for sale in the foyer. Her message of self-acceptance, self-determination and self-love found expression in everything she said: 'You have to come to terms with yourself exactly as you are'; 'No one can fulfil you with their love until you fill yourself with love'; 'Everyone is made of love, we are nothing but love'; 'Stop waiting for someone else to come in and switch on the light'.

We were told that self-love is a necessary foundation to the loving of God: 'How can you reject yourself? Then you reject God'; 'You have to accept yourself ... that is your foundation. God is within you'; 'You are an ocean of grace, you are an ocean of love'.

And this 'ocean of love' should be plunged into without expecting anything back. One of her devotees wanted to know whether, if she got her work colleagues to accept her, she would then be able to accept herself. ShantiMayi responded with some straight talking: 'You've got this commodity stuff where you lay down a dollar and want something a little more – you always want a profit. In the spiritual world, whatever we do for our spiritual Self – Realization is whatever it is – that is the profit itself, nothing more. It's not like you're putting all of this in a bank account somewhere ... They [the work colleagues] are your guru, they are your spiritual friends ... they have been sent to your realm just to open your heart. So, you can't get anything out of it. You can't extract any chocolate. There's nothing to get here until you turn it around.'

I had really enjoyed the first session but on the second day ShantiMayi got cross with one of her devotees. 'Will you *ever* put your heart towards me?' she asked, her face flushed and her eyes wide with exasperation. My fragile faith was shaken. How could a guru be enlightened if they got angry? Aren't they supposed to be able to stand back from their emotions, let their anger wash over them? Shouldn't she be 'an ocean of love' for her troubled devotee?

That night I had dinner with Mr Hospitality in the Madras Café. Hans, a fourteen-year devotee of Amma, joined us. He said that Amma had been known to get very angry backstage: 'Sometimes she is *Kali* – destroying the ignorance of the universe with her baleful eyes and big black tongue. Amma changes with different people according to what they need – soft and warm with me, wielding her bloody sword with someone else.'

'Yes, yes,' agreed Mr Hospitality, 'a teacher must be mutable – he should be capable of being as hard as rock, and as soft as water.'

'So how do you know if you've found the right teacher?' I asked, still unsure.

'The only true way is to see if you reach enlightenment, and that can take a long time,' replied Hans. 'In the meantime you must just trust and watch.'

Mr Hospitality told us a story he attributed to Ramakrishna, the nineteenth-century spiritual leader: 'The guru was asked, "What is enlightenment?" Ramakrishna replied, "You are asking this as a drop of water asks the ocean, "Who am I?" The ocean says, "Come closer, jump in." The droplet of water jumps in and the ocean asks, "Now what are you?" The water replies, "I am That. I am You, and yet I am exactly the same as before." In other words, Lucy, you can continue to sit by the side of the ocean and ask questions, or you can jump in and dissolve into the ocean. You are already who you need to be. It's up to you. Yes, yes.'

Hans added, 'You are already That – that which you seek. Seeking, questing, always looking beyond, takes you far from everything that you already are. It's very simple really. We have to come home to ourselves.'

I went back to ShantiMayi the next day wondering if I could dissolve into the ocean and come home to myself. She was certainly on form.

A devotee asked, 'If I open my heart will all of my problems disappear?'

ShantiMayi replied, 'When I was a Park Ranger in Oregon, what I enjoyed about my problems was that they were always there. When I solved one problem another problem would roll right in … I tied myself in knots. And then, one day, I gave up my problems and never had another one. That's a true story.' There was a pause. 'When you go to your heart, things are very clear.'

This was promising stuff. I was over my anger issues and loving the homespun advice and salmon-pink cardies. I would have kept on the ShantiMayi trail except that she was starting a ten-day silent *Vipassana* meditation retreat with her devotees and wouldn't be giving these regular chats for its duration. By the time she was out and talking again I would be travelling to Chennai. I bought a tape recording of one of the *satsangs* and a photograph, however, and determined to look her up on the Internet. Perhaps she did world tours like Amma, although I couldn't imagine her renting out stadiums for marathon hugging sessions.

I only made it to Pankash's morning classes during the ShantiMayi sessions – but my impression of a pony fit for nothing but the knacker's yard grew in accuracy. I put up with it because I was learning a lot about the finer details of my anatomy – I'd never studied the inner workings of my toes, buttocks or eyelashes in such detail before – but I can't say that the classes were a real pleasure, or that they took me to a more peaceful meditative state. I found it quite mechanical and the instructions required too much thought for it to be possible to switch off the *chitta vritti*. It was lacking the flow, the movement of energy, that made it possible to forget myself, at least for a moment or two, which I had really enjoyed in Simon's classes, and latterly with Vinay P. Menon. The only thing that cheered me up every morning was the idea of breakfast at the Madras Café. 'Muesli, toast, south Indian coffee,' said MP as I walked in, more a statement than a question.

At one of these breakfasts I got talking to Julie, an American living in England who spent two months at the Divine Life Society every year, and her friend – Mr Prasad. He had lived in the ashram for twenty-five years but had left it eighteen months ago 'to lead a more independent life'. He was working as a yoga teacher, and many of his students were Westerners. As I was feeling rather over my *Iyengar asana* classes I was quite relieved to hear from Mr Prasad that the real yoga of India runs much deeper.

'For Indians, right from babyhood, yoga is part of everyday life,' he told me. 'Because we sit on the floor, have our squatting toilets and such, we do not have the same physical problems as Westerners. We can start with a higher level.

'In the West *asana* becomes the object, Westerners are driven by dissatisfaction, they become fanatical and want to condition others to their way when the whole point is to decondition, to remove the barriers. We Indians are taught "you are not the body" and "do not desire", but in the West, you *are* the body. The body is all you are, and fulfilment of desire is everything. The Westerners I teach think yoga is purely physical – *asana* and *pranayama; Hatha* yoga only – but yoga is a harmonious way of living. This is the real yoga.'

Mr Prasad tried to expand his students' awareness beyond *asana* and *pranayama*, to embrace all eight of the limbs described in Patanjali's yoga *sutras*. Two of the other limbs, the *yamas* and *niyamas*, I knew about, thanks to the Swoony Swami. Mr Prasad explained the others; *pratyahara* means controlling the senses so that the yogi can be free of the distractions of the outside world. 'Then there is *dharana,* concentration of the mind – one-pointedness. You focus the mind on one point – like pouring oil from one vessel to another. Nothing is lost, there is one unbroken thought. The next step is *dhyana* – meditation. This can only be done when you have mastered *dharana*. But in the end there are many paths, and only one goal – the eighth limb – *samadhi*.' He expounded, in a variation on the Ramakrishna water theme. 'In *samadhi*, you are one with consciousness – you are not an individual any more, there is no more you. The rainwater drops on the Ganga and it does not say I am rain and you are Ganga. The two are one. In *samadhi* you start to see the Self in every living thing.'

He returned to the Western predicament. 'But maybe *asana* is the most suitable start point for the Western mind, which cannot sit and meditate straight away. At least *asana* restores energy to dull bodies and starts to awaken the Self to other possibilities. Some people will go on to the next level.'

I wanted to go on to the next level – and I wanted to do it now. I couldn't see how being shouted at and told to stretch my upper eyelashes was going to get me to the bliss of *samadhi*. Anyway, Mr Prasad told me that 'most ordinary Indians are not practising much *asana* over the age of twenty-five'. He explained that *pranayama* should be the main focus for adults, and over the age of fifty, *dhyana* is the key practice. Was I already too old for my blue sticky mat?

I was keen to ditch the fanatical, dissatisfied Westerner label. I wanted to become an 'ordinary' Indian, living harmoniously, extending my yoga practice beyond my mat, moving onto a higher level. I particularly wanted to make sure I practised the yoga that was most appropriate to the place – when in Rome and all that. 'What about Rishikesh?' I asked Mr Prasad. 'Does Rishikesh have its own brand of yoga?' He explained that 'the yoga of Rishikesh is the age-old yoga of love and devotion – *Bhakti* yoga – this is what we are doing every day.'

As I had seen, beneath its commercial surface, in which the purchase of CDs and OM T-shirts seemed to offer as quick a way to merging with cosmic bliss as sitting atop a mountain, Rishikesh was a simple, old-fashioned place. Whether they wore orange robes or not, everyone was dedicated to the worshipping of God – in any, or all of his thousands of Hindu guises. This, after all, was the 'city of saints', the gateway to the sacred Himalaya, packed with pilgrims, *rishis* and *sadhus* on their way to *samadhi*. This was a very different India to that of Delhi or Pune, or even Amritapuri.

I decided to spend the rest of my time in Rishikesh applying myself to the yoga of devotion. Although I had been there, done it, bought the Hugging Mother's 'Chant Your *Mantra*' stickers, I had enjoyed

ShantiMayi's *Bhakti* yoga *satsangs*. It was clearly a broad church, available in lots of different formats, and Mr Hospitality was happy to assume the role of my *Bhakti* teacher and guide.

The Hidden Saint, an energetic Sivananda devotee, had climbed the mountain behind his tiny house, a journey of 24 kilometres, at 3 a.m. every day for the last sixty years. When people asked if they could join him he would dismissively say, 'You wouldn't be able to keep up.' He was feeding a hundred *sadhus* the next day and invited Mr Hospitality to come along and bring a friend.

Unfortunately only ten *sadhus* turned up, despite the promise of free food, and the Hidden Saint decided to remain hidden, despite what Mr Hospitality called a 'definite and most insistent invitation – yes, yes.' At first it didn't seem to matter that much. Mr Hospitality and I sat in the warm courtyard at the back of the house, in which Sivananda himself had done *tapas* for twelve years, soaking up the sun and the sight of these *sadhus* in their trademark orange. Unusually there was one *sadhu* dressed in black, although he did have an orange shoulder bag, which he'd decorated with pink shiny streamers. And there was one *sadhu* who had trumped all the dress codes – by wearing nothing at all. Mr Hospitality told me that naked *sadhus* tended to have airs of grandeur and think they are one step above those still attached to their clothes. I didn't know quite where to look so I concentrated on eating my lunch – vegetable curry and rice served on an eco-friendly plate made of dried-out leaves, and a delicious rice pudding in a little leaf bowl of its own. When we had finished we fed our bowls to the waiting cow at the gate.

I wanted to take a photograph of these men; they were an arresting sight. Their markings ranged from the three horizontal lines of the *Saivite* to an orange inverted triangle decorated with orange dots, to two vertical lines separated by a slash of red. Their hairstyles were diverse –

there were two with thick black ropes of hair coiled on their heads, just like the *sadhu* at the Sivananda ashram in Kerala, several with frizzy grey matted locks, and lots of orange turbans. Unsurprisingly the naked man refused to be photographed – quite a relief as he wasn't much of a poster boy – but the others seemed amenable. One asked for a blessing for the goddess Lakshmi. How lovely, I thought. Then Mr Hospitality explained that this was his way of asking for money, Lakshmi being the goddess of wealth. I gave him 10 rupees and then they all wanted cash, becoming more belligerent by the second. Time for a sharp exit.

'They wouldn't have behaved that way if the Hidden Saint had been there,' said Mr Hospitality. 'Most disappointing, yes, yes. The ashrams and the monasteries look after them – and as you saw, so does the Hidden Saint, so there is no need to ask for money. They could eat five times a day if they wanted to. Most of them are middle class and well educated so there is really no excuse. Ah well, let us take it as a lesson. As Swami Sivananda himself once said, "Beware of men in orange."'

We agreed to meet again to celebrate 26 January, India's Republic Day and an auspicious bathing day in the *kumbh mela* calendar, with a trip to Haridwar.

Haridwar, meaning 'gateway to the gods', is only an hour's drive from Rishikesh, and is one of the holiest places in India. Legend has it that it is one of only four cities on which gods and demons dropped a few drops of amrita as they wrestled for possession of the *kumbh*, or pot, containing the nectar. This was to be an *ardh kumbh*, marking the halfway point between full *kumbhs*, which happen every twelve years. It would be a good place in which to perform some more yoga of devotion, and we could have a dip in the Ganges and visit some of the city's holiest shrines.

We began at the Maa Mansadevi Temple, billed as one of the most important temples in northern India. *Mansa* means wishes and the Devi or goddess who fulfils these wishes was, unsurprisingly, in demand. We took a three-minute cable car ride to save us a one-hour slog up the Shivalik hills and joined the thousands of Indians on a pilgrimage to the temple. Hands sleeved in orange appeared from every nook and corner of the temple demanding money in return for blessings and *kumkum*. After an hour of being pushed and shoved and bled dry of rupees we finally came face to face with the Mansadevi shrine. To mark this highly auspicious moment, a bad-tempered man in orange snatched away our plastic bags containing our budget-priced offerings to the goddess – coconut slices, tinsel and red plastic bangles that we had purchased outside the temple – and threw them unceremoniously on the ground behind him. Seeing its fate, I was glad we had decided not to go for the full deluxe package – a red-wrapped glitter fest of abundant fruits and 'gold' bangles. Eventually we came face to face with two trees on which were tied thousands of red and yellow threads. We were supposed to tie a thread onto one tree and return to untie one from the same tree once our wish had been fulfilled, but in the din I misunderstood Mr Hospitality's instruction and untied someone else's thread – thereby nullifying both my wish and theirs. I hoped he or she hadn't wished for something really important.

After a depressing lunch break amongst the crumbling buildings, wandering pigs, chickens and aimless beggars of rainy Haridwar central, we made our way through the narrow back streets, past children playing by open drains, through a market lined with multi-coloured hair comb stalls and men demonstrating the virtues of plastic mincers, towards the Ganges. Row upon row of beige tents big enough to house a platoon of scouts lined the river – it looked like a small and rather deso-late town. I had expected to see the place teeming with devotees eager to cleanse away their sins with a dip in the adored holy river, which Hindus believe was sent to earth by King Bhagiratha in order that the ashes of his relatives could be washed of their sins and ascend to heaven. According to Swami Sivananda's book, *Mother Ganges*, things got a bit out of control and the king had to ask Shiva to restrain the river lest it submerge the whole of the earth. Happily Shiva rose to the challenge, receiving the river in his hair and letting it drip over him.

I'd also imagined that the river would be a major draw for the *sadhu* population. I had seen pictures of a full *kumbh mela* on television – apparently drawing a crowd so big it was visible from space. There had been images of *sadhus* smoking clay pipes around fires, clad in nothing much more than grey *vibhuti* ash. They had charged naked and enthusiastic into the choppy waters, brandishing tridents, flags and drums, loudspeakers amplifying their sacred whoops and cries of *'Rama Rama'* and *'Jai Ganga'* as policemen tried to maintain order amongst the overexcited, cheering crowds.

Aside from a lady struggling not to reveal any undergarments as she was immersed, fully clothed, by her husband and sister, and a man with withered legs being given a good-natured dunk by some friends, there was no one else around. Our only company were policemen brandishing sticks at nothing in particular. We walked a little way upriver and found a very pretty spot opposite some fields – a few metres away from a woman washing the lunch dishes, and a couple of cows who were very interested in making their lunch out of my red rose garland. I had no intention of giving it to a cow – I was very attached to it, having bought it for 50 rupees from a tiny little girl with the wise eyes and handknitted headscarf of an eighty-year-old. She had appraised me with an air of great seriousness as she continued to thread her garlands, sitting like a little doll on the family barrow.

There were steps down to the water and a chain to hold onto. Mr Hospitality anointed his own head and moved to a respectful distance. In I plunged – all the way up to my knees. It was absolutely freezing but I managed to stay in for several seconds thanks to an unexpected burst of sunshine that sparkled down on the water and made me burst out laughing. I scooped up the water with both hands and poured it over my head. Droplets the size of diamonds danced in the sunshine and I didn't care that a crowd had gathered to watch the curious white lady in her Brotherhood of the White Robes dress washing away her sins. I tore the roses off the garland, throwing them one by one into the water, as I watched Mother Ganges pull them inexorably downstream. The cows looked on mournfully. The Ganges's peaceful, calming and happy effect on me was undeniable. I remembered what Sonu, the proud owner of a small CD shop opposite the Madras Café, told me: 'I am liking Ganga very much. I like to sit and peace my mind. If I have a headache or too much music in the shop, someone is asking me "play *mantras*, play Krishna Das, play Deva Premal", I go to the Ganga and it's "aahh, Shanti". I smell the moss and empty my mind.'

Next stop was the nearby ashram of Shri Shri Ma Anandamayee, 'the Blissful Mother', born in East Bengal in 1896. A passing sage discovered her when she was just nine months old. He declared her 'Mother Incarnate' and set in motion a precocious career in which, like Amma, she spent her childhood singing the Lord's name, talking to plants, animals and invisible beings, going into trances, having fits in which her body shape became distorted, and burning the family's dinner. She would later claim that she was fully conscious of her Eternal Self from birth. She was married at the age of thirteen, to Bholonath, but the couple never consummated the relationship. When sexual thoughts occurred to her husband, her body would stiffen and she would give him spontaneous electrical shocks. He hoped that the situation would be temporary but it turned out to be permanent, and, in 1922, ignoring his family's calls that he find a new wife, he was initiated as one of her devotees. Two years after that she stopped feeding herself. Fearing that she would 'leave her body', her devotees, who were by now sizeable in number, fed her themselves. She travelled throughout India from 1932 until her *samadhi* in 1982, and was adored wherever she went. But she refuted the guru tag, saying that she was just 'a little girl'. She was actually a stunningly beautiful woman with long dark hair, high cheekbones and big, brown, gentle eyes that seemed to inhabit a faraway world.

We sat down on the steps to watch the late-afternoon sunshine warm the serene white marble temple containing her *samadhi* shrine. An old man in orange robes shuffled around the corner. He had the pale, papery skin of the very old, a slight stoop, a strong hook nose and beady eyes. He walked with difficulty, owing to a nasty burn on his leg; his orange socks and bandages drooped around his white shins.

Mr Hospitality's face lit up. 'Swami Vijayananda,' he whispered to me conspiratorially. 'I last saw him ten years ago and I never thought I'd see him again.'

'Let us sit for a while,' said the old man. As he distributed oranges to the small crowd that had gathered before him he told us how he had come to India in search of spiritual guidance at the age of thirty-six. When he'd left his medical practice in France where he was earning good money his neighbours had shaken their heads and said, 'There must be a woman involved.' Which, in the end, there was. He had met 'Ma' for the first time at six o'clock in the evening on 2 February 1951 at her ashram in the holy city of Varanasi – a moment that he later described as 'like somebody throwing a lighted match in gun-powder'. A few hours later, in his hotel room, he realized that he had found the guru he was looking for. It was love, but not the worldly love that ends in disillusionment and sorrow. This was the infinite divine love felt between a guru and a devotee – 'the radiance of love, a love pure and luminous', capable of liberating him from worldly attachments. He never went back to France.

Keen to find out if Mr Prasad's point of view on yoga in India was a common one, I asked him whether he still practised *asana*. 'When I was young it was very rare to meet someone who had any understanding of yoga or spirituality. Now there are many people interested in this. It is, 'ow you say, "new age". I did practise when I first came to India but not now – I am eighty-nine, you know. I had a master with whom I studied. I practised every day. But you know, *asana* is very secondary in India to the rest of yoga. In the West it is the first and only concern but here this is not the case. Many Indians do practise yoga, especially the educated Indians, but not like the West – here it is less *asana*. For them it is unremarkable. It is a habit, at home, on their own.'

'A bit like my father's gin and tonic at the end of the day?' I wondered.

Swami Vijayanada laughed. 'Perhaps. Other things beside *asana* are important to Indians – a vegetarian diet is important for lightness and *ahimsa*. But in the West it is so cold they must eat meat.' He ate another slice of orange thoughtfully. 'But slowly the West is turning. There is more understanding of the way animals are treated and killed. Buddha ate meat, you know, but only animals which had not been killed specifically for eating – they had died of old age or had an accident.'

'Were there a lot of accidents in Buddha's time?' someone asked.

Everyone, including Swami Vijayananda, laughed.

We spent another hour with the charming *swami*, sitting in a line on the marble steps, watching ever-longer shadows falling over Ma's *samadhi mandir*. We didn't want to leave but the sun was setting on our day of devotion to the Divine and my still-wet hair was making me shiver. The Ganges dip had been exhilarating and Swami Vijayananda's peacefulness and gentle wit were a welcome tonic after the 'money for wishes' experience of the Maa Mansadevi Temple.

Caroline had explained to me that in *Advaita Vedanta*, the foremost strand of Hindu philosophy, the Divine is believed to be everywhere and in everything. I had to admit that this concept had never regained the air of utter straightforwardness that it had seemed to possess under the stars in Turkey but getting in touch with it certainly seemed to be easier here, in Rishikesh and Haridwar, than elsewhere. It seemed to me that MP and Mr Hospitality had that quality, as if there was something unshakeable, a bright, shimmering quality, which lit them from within. I loved the idea that I was made of the same stuff as them – that my *atman*, my Eternal Self, was in essence *brahman*, universal cosmic consciousness. I had never been able to get to grips with the dualistic view of the Divine as something totally distinct from me. It made me feel small and lonely. I found it something of a relief, a weight off my shoulders, to think that my Self was part of something much bigger, and that I wasn't in this thing on my own.

I decided to devote my last day in Rishikesh to another kind of *Bhakti* yoga: watching the rich shower love and devotion on their favourite deity – money. I hired a driver to take me up to Vinay P. Menon's place of work – 'Ananada in the Himalayas', half an hour and several leagues of luxury away from the Great Ganga.

I had been expecting great things of this five-star spa but I hadn't anticipated that the journey, along a winding road cut into the forested foothills of the Himalaya, would be so breathtaking. Akhil, my driver, took every hairpin bend with great gusto, hurtling past big yellow signs – 'After whisky driving risky' and 'Life is joyful, live to see it' – as he scattered families of monkeys playing in the middle of the road. Eagles soared overhead, coming to rest in families of three, perching on a branch to enjoy the rich, green and woolly forest carpet made hazy by the morning sunshine. Rishikesh lay quietly in the valley below, protected by the ribbon of holy river, silenced at last by the distance between us.

Vinay came to meet me in the yellow and blue Viceregal Tea Lounge, where life-sized portraits of the former Maharajah of Tehri Garhwal, Lord Mountbatten and Mrs Indira Gandhi hung overlooking the rose gardens. He showed me the oldest billiards table in India – a witness to 'some of the most famous political personages' – the chandeliered Viceregal Hall, previously the Maharajah's skating rink, and the Viceregal Suite with its own wraparound terrace, four-poster bed, telescope, private Jacuzzi and personal member of staff.

We jumped in a white buggy and zoomed at breathtaking speed towards the modern spa. A stone Ganesh garlanded with orange flowers greeted us, bowls of pink petals decorated every table surface and intricate wall-mounted geometric *Tantric yantras* with golden inlays depicted cosmic unity. Vinay took me on a tour, proudly showing off huge sunken baths from which to gaze at the mountains, the shallow pool with pebbles from the Ganges around which the sauna-bound walked seven times in a clockwise direction, and the rich brass pot used for trickling luke-warm herbal oil over the third eye in the luscious *Sirodhara* treatment.

'What a wonderful smell,' I remarked to Vinay – I was reminded of the rose garden next to the Viceregal Palace.

'Actually, ma'am,' he replied, 'we are calling it "aroma".'

He showed me the different venues that his students, the likes of Melinda Gates and the Barclay brothers, could choose for their private yoga sessions. There was the eight-columned music belvedere where Zoë Williams had her lesson, an amphitheatre, a wood-lined sunroom in the Viceregal Palace and my favourite – the terrace overlooking the sal and ancient mango trees, outside the simple room dedicated to Shri Shri Ma Anandamayee. The official Ananda story is that she lived in the room for twenty-five years but Akhil told me that she had only visited it occasionally, sometimes to give *darshan* to the Maharajah and once to give an audience to Mrs Indira Gandhi. Whatever the truth, the room itself, and the terrace, had a stillness that reached towards the Himalaya in the far distance.

Unable to spend £150 on a standard room for the night I contented myself with lunch – including a quick stop-off in the Pavilion bar. I stood and stared at the top-of-the-range spirits and bottles of French wine on proud display. My own spirits soared.

Seeing the look in my eye, Vinay gently nudged me out of the room. 'But ma'am, this is place people are coming for reasons of health and all, and we are not encouraging our guests to drink.'

The bar was in fact deserted, and I hadn't quite reached the point of being prepared to drink alone. As I settled down to lunch in the Tree

Tops restaurant I congratulated myself on my *saucha* – my purity of mind and body – adding another day to the Edge family record of thirty-four days without a drink. And then – the man at the next table cracked open an ice-cold tin of Heineken. I watched transfixed as he poured the amber liquid into his glass.

I surrendered to the moment, immediately and completely, and ordered two. I was pissed as a fart within five minutes. Actually, this was rather handy, as I was finding it hard to relax amongst the starchy tablecloths and starchy waiters. In fact, everyone (except Vinay) was a bit starchy – especially the guests. No one smiled or laughed. Perhaps they were all miserable because of the diets they had been prescribed, I thought, but the food – fish tikka and the unlikely combination of guava ice cream on a bed of grated carrots cooked in milk – was delicious, even though it was low fat. No, I think they were just having trouble with the recognition that they were paying top dollar to live in paradise and still weren't happy.

I realized I was actually quite enjoying the simple life. I was getting used to sitting on hard ashram floors for long periods of time, singing along to the beat of the *tabla*, or a guitar, sitting on the banks of the Ganges watching the great river rush downhill purifying every-thing in its path, and wearing crap clothes that hid my body shape. I hadn't managed to surrender the comforts of my room at the Great Ganga, or surrender my make-up to the universe, but I had spent nearly three weeks in Rishikesh wandering about in a woollen poncho down to my knees, a green plastic mac and a beanie hat, my forehead a big smudge of temple *kumkum*. I was definitely letting myself go, and it felt good.

I met Mr Hospitality for one last meal at the Madras Café. Rain lashed down and the power failed, the generator hummed and we shared a Himalayan Health Pilau and *Paneer* Tikka Masala as the windows steamed up. MP gave me a going-away present – a traveller's bag complete with secret pockets and an embroidered symbol that would ward off evil. I cried into my final coconut and raisin rice pudding, on Mr Hospitality's shoulder and finally into my pillow that night.

I left simple, old-fashioned Rishikesh having chosen the Madras Café as my temple and the devoted MP and Mr Hospitality as my deities. I could feel pleased with my own level of devotion – I had visited the café twice a day, come rain or hail stones, for the last three weeks. Perhaps I had, after all, experienced the real yoga of Rishikesh.

~ 11 ~

'A hump is there,
like a camel'

I left Rishikesh as I had arrived – in pitch-darkness. The Ambassador made its slow, uncertain way through the early-morning fog, passing the shadowy forms of cows and cyclists, towards Haridwar train station. I arrived to find what I thought was a mass of cloth piled high on the platform. And then the cloth started to move – coaxed into human form by the light. Whole families had been sleeping on the station floor. Eventually these, the station's permanent residents, made way for its more temporary occupants, lining the back wall as if they were an audience about to watch a performance. The opening scene must have been a familiar one to them – the *chai* stalls doing steady business at 3 rupees a mug, teenage girls and men with two tummies trying to have a private audience with the metre-wide display of the red scales, and the porters staking out wealthy-looking Indian businessmen and mothers with their hands full of children.

Once we were aboard the train the *chai* stream turned into a river, flowing up and down the aisle, carrying with it plastic washing-up bowls that bobbed up and down to cries of 'chip', 'bisceet', 'chocolat'. Breakfast was a choice of vegetable cutlet or non-vegetarian omelette, served with two slices of white bread wrapped in smiley face paper, which advised me to 'Eat Pure … Be Sure'. The train made very slow progress, crawling along 260 kilometres of track, eventually coming to a halt outside Delhi station six hours later. Several businessmen, with urgent appointments and important briefcases, jumped off the train and impatiently walked up the tracks.

As soon as the train reached the platform all hell broke loose. None of the passengers could get off the train because the porters, in their red and gold heraldry, had launched an invasion. Jammed between aunties, children and irate businessmen, I saw my suitcase, which I had been told to store at the opposite end of the carriage, being lifted high and away. 'Stop, thief!' I cried but my voice was drowned out in the pandemonium. It took me so long to get to the platform that I was quite convinced I would never see the suitcase again, so when I spotted it on the head of a porter, I was delighted. The delight quickly turned to anger as his partner-in-crime, a smooth-talking bully, outlined his terms and conditions – 100 rupees for the porter and another 500 rupees for a taxi into town. I refused to pay and the porter refused to put my case down. The Mexican stand-off lasted for several minutes. It became clear that the only way I was going to get my hands on my bag again would be to pay the porter. But I sure as hell wasn't going to be charged 500 rupees for a journey of 3 kilometres. As soon as he put the suitcase down I thrust the porterage money in his hand and charged off to the pre-paid rickshaw stand. Unfortunately my case slowed me down and the by now baying crowd, all angry eyes and threatening body language, surrounded me – the hunted animal. I would like to claim that I simply smiled in the face of adversity, took a few yogic breaths and watched the crowd part before me as it felt my peaceful vibrations. This would be a lie. What I said actually, screamed actually, at the top of my voice actually, was, 'I don't want a fucking taxi. Fuck off and leave me alone.' So much for *ahimsa* – non-violence. The Swoony Swami would have been disappointed in me, and worried about the boomerang effect of such an outburst, but it did at least have the effect of creating a moment of disorientation – as a rough translation was passed around the crowd. In this gap I managed to buy a coupon for a 32-rupee ride to Karol Bargh and jump in a waiting rickshaw.

Delhi was on a deadline. In its rush to modernize, it couldn't pause for breath – it was too busy throwing flyovers and skyscrapers into the air and extending the foundations of its new metro. I felt very small as I sat in that tiny rickshaw, breathing in the fumes of a three-lane highway. The contrast to peaceful, old-fashioned Rishikesh could not have been greater. I missed the clean air, the protection of the Himalaya beyond the town, MP's good nature and the friendship of Mr Hospitality. I needed a refuge while I waited for my train to Chennai. One of the Divine Lifers had told me about the Angan Vegetarian Restaurant in Karol Bagh; he thought it was Delhi's answer to the Madras Café. It would be a good place to have lunch and rest up before boarding the 18.40 GT Express for Chennai, a journey of thirty-six hours – if it was on time.

As the rickshaw left the busy, polluted streets and turned into Karol Bagh, I began to relax; here was evidence of a slower pace, an older Delhi. I asked the rickshaw driver to drop me on the corner of a street market that was in full swing – *lungis* were displayed alongside American-brand sweatpants and children's nylon party dresses in bright pink and primrose yellow. The charms of gaudy handbags and bangles were demonstrated on the arms of tiny girls, wandering wallahs in training. Their brothers' waists were too small to show off the belts that they were selling so these were also carried on their arms – looped like giant leather bracelets. With the guidance of a map given to me by the Divine Lifer I turned off into another side road and picked my way through a street lined with motor mechanic stalls, spare parts piled high on the pavement, and dismembered cars.

And there was Angan's. All of human life was stuffed into its banquette seats —families of eight struggled to contain themselves, surplus babies and octogenarians spilling over into the narrow walkway. The menu spanned from north to south India, and then branched out towards China, America and Italy. I settled on a south Indian *thali* and a 'Bikano Honey Moon' ice cream sundae.

I was soon joined by the suited and booted twenty-something manager of one of the many budget-priced hotels in the area. Joseph introduced himself. It turned out that he had been practising yoga since he was thirteen at an ashram in Kerala and then at a seminary in Agra until he was twenty-one. 'I am Catholic and very flexible but I did not want to be a monk, I wanted normal life.' In his opinion, 'many people are thinking yoga is only for Hindus so Christians and Muslims don't do. But Jesus was in the Himalaya and he was talking to people as he sat in lotus position.'

We talked about the Western interest in yoga, which had hit his hometown of Kovalam, a touristy beach resort in far away Kerala. Joseph told me that 'now when I go home I see yoga class on beach for Westerners. I am getting worried – they are not doing correctly.' He imitated someone throwing his or her arms about in wild abandon. 'I am worried they hurt themselves – they have to keep breath and timing otherwise yoga become gyminations. Lino Miele, he is Italian Ashtanga teacher, coming every year Kovalam. Many Westerner student come but very expensive. Why Westerner don't like Indian teacher?' I ventured that some do – that I was on my way to see T.K.V. Desikachar in Chennai, but that some Westerners prefer to follow their regular teachers to India, and perhaps others, who would like to study with an Indian teacher, find it hard to find one who will teach them in a way that has enough familiar anchor points.

I asked him whether he knew of many Indians practising *asana*. He replied that 'in city young womans go gyminations and beauty parlour, in the Western way. *Asana* class can be glamour fitness for young rich womans wanting Western influence and all.' I told him about *Elle* India's January edition that had featured Deepika Mehta, yoga instructor, in its 'Leading Ladies' feature, alongside a DJ, a model and a designer. She was teaching 'power yoga', a combination of *Ashtanga*, Pilates and jazz ballet, to packed classes in Mumbai, commenting that 'even though yoga is of Indian origin it's sad that I've had to learn it through the West'.

'This article is correct,' agreed Joseph. 'It is most unfortunate making that yoga is back coming through Western dominance, but on balance I am pleasing that young Indian womans are some *asana* doing.' He paused, looking thoughtful. 'It is a matter of fact that many older Indian womans are not importance giving to exercise – if Indian womans are wealthy they are fattening. They are maybe *Hatha* yoga doing at home – some gentle *asana* and *pranayama* – but they are not everyday class going, not like Westerners. They are more following the devotional *Bhakti* yoga – everyday Indian middle-class womans is doing *puja* for her husband and children.'

'What about the poor?' I asked Joseph. 'Do they practise any kind of yoga?'

'In village poor womans don't go anywhere, working very hard always, enough physical work – no need for *asana*. A lot of womans are breaking rocks. Their husbands may be drinking.'

I had seen these tiny women, their skins blackened and hardened by the sun, working on building sites and carrying lumps of concrete on their heads. Not only did they spend all day shifting concrete, they did all the housework, too. They were far too busy trying to survive to unroll a blue sticky mat, even if they could have afforded one.

I asked him whether he still practised. 'I am like all Indian men; I am very tired with business. When we men should be yoga we are on train – modern life means no yoga. Yoga must be every day – you must rise before sunrise, do your daily bathroom parts and then *puja* and *asana*. There are fixed timings for everything – if you do yoga as daily life you don't need doctor. It is part of daily life but in our modern life we cannot do because we have to work.'

A well-spoken and handsome government official with whom I shared the long journey to Chennai echoed this point of view.

Kedarnath put down his copy of Salman Rushdie's *Fury* and, curling his toes in his flip-flops, explained, 'We are not practising our yoga in big classes in the Western way. Some Indian people have the guidance of a teacher but classes are small, or for the bespoke individual. We are more likely practising our yoga at home – we are doing very little *asana* and more meditation – and we are breathing and doing *puja*. We are using yoga in the mental way, for clear seeing, and choosing wisely. It is part of our daily life – when work is not getting in the way. I myself am practising headstand like our Mr Nehru – every evening I am coming home and upside downing. Then I am drinking gin and tonic in the Western way.'

I wondered if I would ever persuade my father to precede his evening gin and tonic with some 'upside downing'. It seemed unlikely.

Kedarnath continued. 'Of course, most teenagers are doing only yoga as an extra-curricular activity in school and then dropping. There is not enough time with work and all.'

I told him about my month-long course in Chennai. He replied thoughtfully, stroking his beard. 'Before the West became interested in yoga we were taking it for granted, but now the West has created a new market for yoga in India. Maximum thirty per cent Indian is doing yoga but only one per cent is serious practitioner. Some peoples are making good money out of yoga – teaching to foreigners and the like. Many commercial opportunities present themselves to the astute. Selling yoga to Westerners is big business for us now.'

I would have liked to continue this topic of conversation but Kedarnath was keen to move on to the politics of Noam Chomsky. 'He is leading American intellectual dissident. Have you read this collection of his essays, Lucy?' He pulled out a thick tome. I had to confess that I hadn't. I had read yoga books for the last year, and had only just put them down in favour of *A Suitable Boy*. 'Ahh, Vikram Seth – truly a most scintillating read,' he said appreciatively. Before long he was back on the politics of Noam Chomsky: 'Actually George Bush is as much fundamentalist as Saddam Hussein. The Britisher knows this but the American does not. He does not understand that the war in Iraq was about oil.'

Middle-class Indians take politics very seriously and there had been a number of occasions over the last few weeks in which I wished that I had read more widely. He had more luck engaging me on the painful subject of caste. I had seen lots of marginalized people, *harijans* or *dalits*, on my travels but had been so far unable to turn a blind eye, to shrug my shoulders and reason that it was simply these poor people's karma, their destiny to be 'Untouchable', believed to pollute everything they touched. I agreed wholeheartedly when he remarked that 'the caste system is one of the truly last and most unwanted symbols of fiefdom – I abhor it. It must be banished from our kingdom.' I was glad that the political importance of this underclass was growing and that they could no longer be ignored.

We were interrupted in the middle of this conversation by the arrival of the resplendent Fat Controller and his even fatter wife. Following a discussion in English in which it was established that the new arrival held a senior position arranging the distribution of raw materials within the railway, he was henceforth treated with the kind of respect normally reserved for a 'Britisher' royal. He looked like a member of the landed gentry in his tweed jacket, shirt, tie and polished shoes – the only difference was the yellow sapphire on his right-hand index finger. Such was the weight of their presence that Kedarnarth and I felt it incumbent upon ourselves to move out of the carriage; he moved into the one adjacent, which fortuitously was empty, and I took a window seat in the corridor. The next twenty-four hours passed in a steady alternation of heavy snores (his and hers) and phone calls – hers in Hindi to assorted family members, and his in English, to his stockbroker.

I distracted myself with *A Suitable Boy* and watching the passing countryside through double-thickness, double-dirty windows that cast a yellow haze over the fields of central India. I saw some scenes in close-up – endless pampas grass, orchards, oranges piled high in washing-up bowls, goatherds with their flocks, schoolgirls in pressed shirts and pleated skirts, their hair bouncing excitedly in skipping-rope plaits as they played, buffalo pulling carts along the road, tiny huts heaving with huge families. But most of the views out of the window were long shots, far away forests and mountains, which I couldn't identify in my guide book, distant places I would never visit. I was desperate to climb into one of these views, to fill my lungs with fresh forest air but I couldn't even open the windows. I was trapped inside, forcefed the nasty smell of sour fried food mixed with the Fat Controller's body odour.

By night the four of us had to move back into the same sleeping compartment. I didn't get much sleep and woke to find a cockroach nestled up by my ear. By the time the train pulled into Chennai in the early hours of Sunday morning I was gasping for breath. When we were finally allowed to open the doors I leapt off the train as fast as my suit-case would allow me and stood there conducting my own informal *pranayama* class right there on the platform. Nobody took any notice – Chennai is primarily a business hub and everyone had something more important to do than stand around staring at a hyperventilating Westerner. Nonetheless I felt a small thrill in my stomach alongside the heaving in my lungs; here I was in sprawling Chennai, the capital of Tamil Nadu, the tropical south-eastern state, home to 4 million people and one living yogic legend.

I had to be at the Krishnamacharya Yoga Mandiram (KYM) for the 4 p.m. induction. It was on the other side of town but I had left plenty of time and it was, at least on the map, a straightforward route down the main road. After the obligatory rickshaw driver geography conference outside my hotel we sped off. A U-turn across a dual carriageway was followed by a sharp left into a wide road lined with tailors and silk shops, expensive jewellers and a department store. As usual poverty was never far away. We passed over a stinky bridge, underneath which were slums with battered blue tarpaulin walls, and drew up alongside a beggar with stumps for legs sitting on a homemade trolley, staking out the stationary traffic at the lights. I gave him 100 rupees and he looked as if he'd just won the lottery. I never got used to these haunting spectres during the whole of my time in India, and I never established any set rules of personal conduct. My behaviour was erratic; sometimes I gave a few rupees, at other times 100; sometimes I gave nothing, or turned and looked the other way when it seemed that giving everything was not enough, so giving nothing was easier. And then I would feel ashamed of myself and go into financial overdrive at the next opportunity.

Remarkably we arrived at the Mandiram, tucked away in a peaceful side road, fifteen minutes after we left the hotel. There were no hitches, despite a series of twists and turns that bore no resemblance to the straight line of the map. My spirits were high and the sky was the deep blue of an unshakeable south Indian winter. No more Rishikesh rain – and no more yoga teachers with eyelash issues. Desikachar was the current head of a yoga family dynasty that stretched back many centuries, the school was recognized as one of the best in the world and I was just about to meet forty fellow-seekers from every corner of the globe. Yoga school didn't get any better than this.

There were already thirty pairs of Birkenstocks and their imitators outside the school. The line of sandals was so impeccably straight it looked as if it had been made with a measuring stick – but it was simply the keen eye of the school guard, who made it his job to practise the yoga of shoe alignment every day. I made my way past traditional Tamil *kolams* – geometric symbols of protection and good fortune – drawn with chalk dust on the ground, and received a welcome garland of white flowers from graceful, modest women in elegant saris of emerald-green and sapphire-blue.

I stood on the veranda opposite a garlanded black icon of Patanjali and made nervous small talk with some of my fellow students. There were a lot of yoga teachers on the course. Liv and Johan had both been teaching for a while – they'd recently signed up to work for a Swedish company that would be bringing ayurveda, yoga and meditation to stressed-out executives. Roxanne had a thriving business on the other side of the world, teaching ten classes a week and giving massage to Sydney-siders who wanted to stretch an extra inch across their surfboards and yoga mats. Savannah, who was feeling very homesick for her husband and two children back home in Arkansas, had a busy yoga studio and often brought Desikachar's son Kausthub over to the States for workshops. David, teacher of yoga and creative writing, had written a book on how yoga helps creativity flow. His wife was also a yoga teacher and a naturopath. In fact, there were only three of us in this cluster group who weren't yoga teachers. Beckle was a carpenter from Brooklyn and Harley had just given up his job in Silicon Valley to spend a year composing music and studying yoga in Chennai.

We were sent upstairs to a hut-like room thatched with *keet* where the sun filtered through the diamond slats in the bamboo walls, casting geometric shadows over the patchwork quilt of terracotta, orange, brown and red *dhurries*, the thick rugs that softened the floor. A white-bearded and smiling Sri Tirumalai Krishnamacharya – Desikachar's father – his hands in prayer position, cast blessings over the proceedings from a very large black-and-white photograph garlanded with yellow flowers that hung on the wall at the front of the room. Soon the room was full of students – ages ranging from twenty-five to sixty-five years old. Everybody smiled and seemed relaxed; I think we all felt warm and safe, hermetically sealed off from the outside world, bar the sounds of children playing in the street below and chatting mynah birds.

The heads of school sat at the front of the room on pale-blue plastic chairs. T.K.V. Desikachar, henceforward known as 'Sir', and Mr Sridharan, the school's managing trustee and Sir's friend of twenty-five years, wore matching white linen *veshtis* and short-sleeved shirts with pens sticking out of their top pockets, but their physical opposition gave them something of the air of a comedy duo in the tradition of Little and Large, Abbott and Costello or Morecambe and Wise. Sir was the shorter man, with huge bushy eyebrows, neatly parted thick grey hair, a hawkish nose and keen, twinkling eyes behind square-framed glasses. Mr Sridharan's glasses were frameless and oval, his eyebrows indiscernible and his head as bald and smooth as an egg, an egg with soulful kind eyes sitting atop a beanpole.

Mr Sridharan, known affectionately as 'The Boss', explained that the school was run as a *'sanga'*, working together 'for the service of humanity' in a non-profit-making capacity. Apparently the Boss worked without pay, as did Dr P. Jeyachandran – 'he is rich in knowledge and poor in bank account' – giving the money he received from the Indian government, for his work with special needs children, to KYM.

The healing power of yoga had been written into the family DNA a long time ago. Sri Tirumalai Krishnamacharya was born in 1888 into a distinguished family that traced its roots back to the ninth-century yogi and Saint Nathamuni, author of the *Yoga Rahasya* or the 'Secrets of Yoga', a classic text on yoga as a therapeutic tool. He spent his teens studying the *Vedas*, *Sanskrit* and *Sankhya* – the *darshana* or philosophical basis for the practice of yoga – and had lived in the Himalaya for nearly eight years, with yogi Sri Ramamohan Brahmachari, who eventually sent him back down from the mountain to spread the message of yoga's ability to heal. I'd read in *Sri T. Krishnamacharya: The Legend Lives On* that he'd said, 'Yoga is like surgery without instruments.' To increase the healing power of yoga, Krishnamacharya championed the practice of a more diverse range of yoga *asana* – until this point most Indian *asana* were variations on the basic cross-legged sitting poses used for meditation.

Ironically, given his deeply conservative Brahmin upbringing and yoga lineage, Krishnamacharya was responsible for several seismic shifts in the way in which yoga was taught, creating what Georg Feuerstein, author of more than thirty yoga books, calls 'a *Hatha* yoga renaissance in modern times'. Where once yoga was a largely sectarian practice – mainly the province of high-caste initiated Indian men – he began to teach the lay people who came to Mysore to meet him, even women. One of the first was a Latvian called Zhenia Lubanskaia, whom he taught, perhaps unwillingly at first, at the request of his patron, the Maharaja. Indra Devi, as Zhenia became known, was one of the first to export his yoga to the West – arriving in Hollywood in 1947 to teach Marilyn Monroe, Greta Garbo and Gloria Swanson, amongst others.

Iyengar launched his international career with visits to Switzerland, London and Paris in the fifties – a tour arranged by his student Yehudi Menuhin – and the travelling tradition continues to this day. Pattabhi Jois, celebrating his ninetieth birthday in July 2005, still goes on world tours that would exhaust men half his age, his gigs attended by Willem Dafoe, Christy Turlington, Demi Moore, Sting, Madonna and Gwyneth Paltrow.

As well as broadening the base of yoga from a few *asana* to many, from East to West, from sectarian to lay practitioners and from men to women, Krishnamacharya's other huge and unique contribution to the landscape of modern-day yoga was his latter-day belief that it should be adapted to the needs of the individual, an approach that his son has championed. Krishnamacharya urged his pupils to 'teach what is inside you, not as it applies to you, to yourself, but as it applies to the other'. Desikachar fervently believed that there should be no 'one size fits all' approach at KYM – consequently there was no set practice beyond an emphasis on moving with the breath, and lengthening that breath.

Krishnamacharya's yogic DNA had been passed down through Desikachar to his children. Kausthub, an affable, rotund twenty-eight-year-old, was KYM's chief executive, the international face of the

Desikachar empire and our 'Asana Theory' teacher. His big-eyed younger sister Mekhala was very much her father's daughter. She was also an engineering graduate, only just returned from the US college at which she had studied. She would be one of four leading our daily *asana* practice. Their mother Menaka would lead the afternoon 'Application of Yoga' class; she was a handsome, flirtatious woman with a great sense of humour and a fine line in saris – we would never see her in the same one twice.

Kausthub's daughter, a baby dressed in purple satin, spent the afternoon determinedly crawling across the floor, one arm outstretched, trying to reach her beloved grandfather. I wondered what she would grow up to be. Perhaps she would write *Yoga Sutras II* – the long awaited sequel. Maybe she would rebel and run away to Bollywood.

Suddenly it was our turn to take the mike. One by one we came up to the front to introduce ourselves and to receive a rose, a hessian bag packed with 5 kilos of KYM books and CDs, and our very own soft orange *dhurrie*, which we would have with us all day – eventually becoming as attached to it as a child to a comfort blanket, even falling asleep on it during the long hot lunch breaks. These *dhurries* made me feel a long way from the yoga schools of London – no Nuala yoga bags or sticky blue mats here.

The forty students had come to KYM in quite different ways: 'I read about the Yoga Mandiram on the Internet in a Tokyo shopping mall'; 'I read Sri Desikachar's *The Heart of Yoga* and had to come'; 'I was recommended by my teacher in Stockholm'; 'Yoga helped me recover from breast cancer'.

Everyone felt that they had come to the right place: 'I feel as if I have journeyed to the heart of yoga'; 'I wanted to be here in India, studying at the feet of Sir, soaking up all of these great yoga traditions'; 'I am in Chennai simply to find the best *masala dosa*'.

Given that most were body-workers – there were twenty-seven yoga teachers and most of the rest were allopaths, homeopaths, naturopaths and osteopaths – they could have been unbearably smug, but there was little sign of any big egos and thank god, most of them, especially the American seeking the perfect *masala dosa*, seemed to have a sense of humour.

I felt a flutter of excitement as we packed up for the day. In this place, 'the heart of yoga', with teachers directly descended from an ancient yogic sage, on these soft orange *dhurries*, with these like-minded seekers, I was bound to make some progress. I would study the *sutras*, understand how to use yoga to heal, stand on my head without the support of a wall and work towards *chitta vritti nirodhah*. I would try once again to strip away the layers of ego, to become a grain of salt in the Ramakrishna ocean of bliss.

Being at school as a grown-up was just like being at school as a child. We sat on the floor at tiny wooden desks, our *dhurries* rolled up beneath us. We quickly found our places and guarded them jealously. Beckle spent the whole of the first week asleep at the back of the class – he'd been working hard to finish a job for a very rich client before he left and was suffering from exhaustion and jet lag. Savannah, Harley and I sat just in front of him, and Liv and Johan in front of us. As for ten-year-olds, so for grown ups – the front row still contained the highest concentration of question-askers.

Like ten-year-olds we all had our favourite teachers. Kausthub, animated in blue polo shirt and beige chinos, was easy to imagine at the nineteenth hole, though he professed to hate golf. He was popular with everyone, partly because he told lots of jokes: 'How many yoga students does it take to change a light bulb? One but he needs two bricks, three chairs, four bolsters, five blankets and six ropes.'

The Boss was also popular, although his class could not have been in greater contrast to Kausthub's. Looking elegant in a crisp white *veshti* and a grey shirt with two pens in his top pocket, he quickly settled into a teaching style heavy with information. We began the first 'Yoga Philosophy' class with the origins of yoga. Yoga got its first mention in the Indian scriptures *The Vedas* – 'the source of knowledge in ancient India'. He told us that the *sutras* were codified by Patanjali (and now I really did feel as if I were a ten-year-old being told a story) who descended to earth with the neck and head of a snake and the body of a human being. He was a servant of Lord Vishnu, preserver of the universe, who sent him to earth to end man's suffering. He gave three solutions to this suffering – yoga for the mind, ayurveda for the body and Sanskrit grammar for speech.

Over the next couple of days the Boss expounded on the purpose of yoga. He explained that 'the mental plane has five states', the first two of which were all too familiar to me.

Ksiptam is the ten-year-old's predominant state of mind – 'a state of high agitation' in which the mind is like a butterfly. 'In this state we cannot do *asana* or chant, although we may be able to listen to chants.' *Mudham* is the second state – the official state of the blues in which 'the mind is dull, inert and cloudy'. This is the mind state that can so easily descend upon a person if they spend ten hours talking about marge. In the third state – that of *viksiptam* – the mind is able to focus but is concentrating on the activities of doing and thinking rather than on meditation. We should be aiming higher, for *ekagrata,* a state in which the mind is one-pointed and can concentrate, not in ordinary concentration but in a state of higher contemplation. This is a necessary stepping-stone to the fifth state of mind – *niruddham* – 'the objective of yoga' – a state in which the mind sees everything clearly, without the distraction of *chitta vritti*, a state in which the mind is like a 'flawless diamond'. So far so good.

After this, about day three, I entered the confused state of *ksiptam*. My notebooks became a mass of half-finished sentences, crossings-out and question marks. I found it as hard to navigate my way around his lectures as I did to find my way around Chennai. But at least there were maps of Chennai. I couldn't for the life of me work out what the map of his mind, or his teachings, looked like. It was partly his Tamil meets English – 'Tamish' – accent, and partly the way in which his lectures were structured. There were no signposts and we skipped around a lot, moving from sutra II.5 to III.29 to I.27 with seemingly no more logic than that employed by the Chennai Post Office when they changed the house number of the Mandiram from thirteen to twenty-five to thirty-one; apparently they were now considering changing it back to thirteen.

I discussed the problem with my classmates in one of the welcome breaks. We sat on white plastic chairs in the canopied courtyard to the side of the Mandiram and fought the mosquitoes as we sipped fresh coconut juice. The Boss had a lot of fans. How come the others could disentangle Tamish so easily? I think it helped that they were much better acquainted with the *sutras* than me: Savannah taught them to her students in the American south, David and his wife participated in a *sutra* study group; Johan had studied them at home. I took comfort in my *dhurrie* neighbour Harley's frustration – the two of us huddled together to exchange 'I am confused' notes and to read the translation in Sir's *Reflections on Yoga Sutras of Patanjali* – a pretty dog-eared book by the end of the first week. I also tried to take a leaf out of Louise's book; she confessed that she didn't understand much either but she enjoyed his teaching and felt that 'just being around him is being in the presence of yoga'.

I found the afternoon 'Application of Yoga' classes equally baffling. Led by Sir's wife Menaka, we were supposed to observe, assess and plan yoga practices using real-life case studies. Our first case was Louise. She wasn't allowed to say what was wrong with her so the class spent an hour playing an elaborate guessing game in which we observed her, asked her questions to which she could only give brief factual replies, and got her to perform various *asana* that would give us a greater insight into the problem. Menaka aided and abetted us with her questions. 'Can you see tha?' she asked as she pointed at Louise's neck and shoulders. 'You have seen her do *asana,* isn't it. Wha' observation do you have?'

I circled Louise, trying to imitate one who understands what they are looking for – copying the other students' furrowed brows, whispered conferences and thoughtful 'hmms' and 'ahhs'. Everyone else enthusiastically listed Louise's apparent myriad problems on the blackboard – tight hips, a stiff lower back, a stiff upper back, stiff knees and tight hamstrings. It was a wonder she could still walk. Menaka looked doubtful at some of the students' diagnoses and remedial *asana* suggestions but took it all with her customary good humour. Eventually she decided to put us out of our misery. She pointed between Louise's upper shoulder blades and said with a huge smile and a giggle: 'A hump is there, like a camel.'

I had the same trouble understanding body language in Kausthub's '*Asana* Theory' classes. I was never the one he picked to come up to the blackboard to draw a sequence of preparatory poses that would lead to the so-called 'goal pose' – the pinnacle of the practice. Mine was never one of the ten eager hands that shot up when he asked what poses complemented each other: 'Should *bujangasana* counterpose *sarvangasana?*' 'Is *sarvangasana* an effective counterpose to *sirsasana?*' I tried to work it out quietly on my own but my notebook filled with improbable stick men who had lost arms and legs attempting the impossible. The bit of my brain that understood how to shape a one-hour class plan so that it was not in Kausthub's words, 'a never-ending cycle of agony', was missing in action. This lack of natural ability began to get me down. The other students seemed, for the most part, to love it.

The other students' eager questions were often spearheaded by a strong-minded German lady who sat in a commanding position in the front row. Her hand shot up at least once a class, sometimes two or three times. No point, however small, escaped her eagle-eyed scrutiny. The class had more than its fair share of what would, in my schooldays, have

been called Girlie Swots. One Indian-American was an allopath, naturopath and homeopath with a long list of clients. She also managed to
squeeze in a day a week in school and thirty hours of studying. She made
those long days in advertising look like a walk in the park. She was very
driven, telling me, 'I think my mission is to teach people to breathe – I
am going to do some videotapes and maybe some TV. This is my
purpose, and to be a woman.' She was certainly having some success
with the 'be a woman' goal – at least one of the senior students seemed
besotted with her, and she had a man back home.

Thankfully there were also the other classic school typologies. Liv,
with her young elfin face, blonde hair and boho dress sense was the class
babe. There was a touch of the elfin about Christophe, too, but he also
had Mick Jagger lips, dimples and a sexy French accent, and few were
immune to his charms. He took quite a shine to Mrs Desikachar; unfortunately she overheard him saying to Johan that he thought she was very
sexy, but she took it all in her stride and roared with laughter. Harley
was the lovable music geek, spending hours locked away in his apartment composing on his iMac; Roxanne was the fun-loving girl next
door with the Elle Macpherson body and a great line in dirty jokes;
Savannah was the kind one, the class mother, the one we went to when
we had a case of the *mudham* blues; and of course, there was the sporty
one – a golf pro who taught disadvantaged kids back home in Illinois.

There was also a new type – one that had not existed when I was at
school. Johan was the class 'Man About Town'. He very quickly worked
out where the best shops, restaurants and clubs were, noticed when our
outfits colour-matched and was always impeccably groomed. I could
imagine him back home, entertaining friends in his fabulous city apartment – drizzling balsamic vinegar over the strawberries and showing off
his tableware. I shared a rickshaw with him and Liv to school and he
often kept us waiting. It wasn't that he had been out particularly late the
night before, just that he had a lot to do in the morning. He answered his
doorbell with an apologetic, winning smile, wearing nothing but his

dimples and a towel that covered only a small bit of that smooth-skinned body. Somehow I always found it easy to forgive him.

The only classes that weren't punctuated by questions were those in which we weren't supposed to talk, but these carried with them their own frustrations. The day began at 7 a.m. with a one-hour *asana* class. Although most of the school's *asana* work was one to one, they couldn't have found room for forty students to have individual classes every day so we were divided into two groups. The group I was in went to nearby Vedavani, the *Vedic* chanting school, to a room almost identical to the one in the main house and similarly blessed by a photograph of Krishnamacharya.

Geetha Shankar, course administrator and *asana* teacher, gave delicate demonstrations of the postures in her sari – its folds made it difficult to make out the finer points of her breath and *asana* demonstrations, but we were inspired by her grace, ladylike manner and the fact that her spectacles and wavy black hair, caught in a bun, remained in position whatever the pose. Mekhala was our other teacher in the first week. Her US college education sometimes showed through in her choice of grey sweatpants and T-shirts, though she was just as likely to turn up in a *salwar kameez*. Her short, strong, flexible body betrayed her membership of a yoga dynasty – she demonstrated poses effortlessly but without fuss or any apparent ego. She had begun teaching children at the school when she was a child herself, aged twelve. Clearly very bright and focused, she had taught her older brother to chant and we would see her chanting with her father several times over the next four weeks. Although I would have thought this would be terrifying she showed no sign of nerves, always looking calm and centred. Together they taught us what I would call 'Pensioner's Yoga' – every movement was so slow my granny could have done it. We repeated every pose several times, the breath initiating everything.

No need for blue sticky mats here – we weren't moving fast enough to slip. We stood on our soft *dhurries* and raised our hands above our heads on the inhale, lowering them on the exhale. We raised our arms above our heads as we inhaled and tried to touch our foreheads to our shins in *uttanasana* as we exhaled. We inhaled our arms into *virabhadrasana I* or 'warrior I' – one leg bent to 90 degrees, the other straight – and then we exhaled the bent leg straight. Our knees and hands planted on the ground, we arched our backs like cats as we gazed towards our navel and exhaled; inhaling, we moved our spines into deep, smile-shaped curves as we imitated dogs stretching. We lay on our backs, knees bent, and raised our hips off the ground as we inhaled into 'half bridge' or *dvipada pitham*. In *apanasana* we pulled our knees into our chest as we exhaled and moved them slowly away on the inhale. We did everything six times, really slowly – it was as if the ten-minute warm-up in those London classes had been stretched into a full one-hour class. It was curiously exhausting – mentally rather than physically. I longed to leap about, to do something dynamic, anything to escape the snail's pace movements and the escalating *chitta vritti*. Would we ever get going? I found myself longing for the strong shot of coffee served up after class, anything to convince myself I was still alive and kicking. I gulped it down and talked nineteen to the dozen at breakfast time, glad to have escaped the mental torture of the 'slow', 'on the breath', 'just breathe' instructions.

I had to go back to Vedavani later in the morning for *Vedic* chanting classes. Given my chequered history with chanting I had been unsure whether to spend the extra $200 on this optional extra but I felt that progress had been made in Kerala, and at ShantiMayi's *satsangs*, and if there was a chance of experiencing *mudita* again I was going to take it. There was also the strong incentive of the cookies and muffins cooked by children at the Downs Syndrome Association of Tamil Nadu – a day care centre in a northern suburb of Chennai; they delivered two trays of sugary confections to Vedavani every day. If the *Vedic* chanting classes didn't take 'me way to the heavens' as ShantiMayi's *satsangs* had, the muffins surely would.

The chanting classes were very hard work – as one of the senior students told me, '*Vedic* chanting is like going to the gym' – but was worth sticking with because, in Sir's words, '*Vedic* chanting is a purifier'. It requires very precise pronunciation – notated by a sequence of dots and dashes, under and over particular letters. If you get it wrong you can end up wishing hell's fury would rain down upon your favoured guru instead of blessings. It was understandable therefore that Shobana Srinivasan, our teacher, was a perfectionist, especially as we would have to chant before Sir at the closing ceremony: 'You should pronounce in the perfect way'; 'H dot down is there. Aspirate!'; 'Force the letter out'; 'S dot down is there. Retroflex – curl up the tip of your tongue'. The idea was to sing as one voice, without hesitation. Woe betide us if 'doubt is there'.

Despite this perfectionism Shobana was far from a tyrant. In fact, we all loved her, and she was definitely my favourite teacher. We crowded round her in a semi-circle, sitting cross-legged on our rolled-up *dhurries* and competing for her approval; it was just like being in nursery school. It may have been hard work but it was also strangely exhilarating when, after an hour of struggling, we managed to sing, as one voice, '*tapannapamayatanam*', '*naksatranamayatanam*' and '*yassamvathsarasyayatanam*'. It was also, for me at least, my most successful meditation; as with the ShantiMayi chanting sessions, I did manage to forget myself for a moment or two. Not in this case because the chanting sounded like the voices of angels – actually *Vedic* chanting sounds quite hard; it's the German of the chanting world – but because it required such great concentration.

The meditation classes were led by everybody's favourite big sister, Sarawathi, and the maternal Dr Latha Satish, who had an air of the old-fashioned about her – partly to do with her upright stance, glasses and neat bun. We always began with some slow *asana* practice – slower even than the Pensioner's Yoga of the morning sessions, more what might be called 'Nursing Home Yoga'. This seemed the right thing to do, though – it was the end of the afternoon and we were tired and hot. Unfortunately, my *chitta vritti* would always start up again as soon as we began *pranayama*.

I had not made much progress in this area since I'd arrived in India. I was always losing count of the number of breaths, getting distracted by the mosquitoes around my ankles, the blast of the fans on my neck and the building work outside the school. Or I would start off gung-ho – holding my breath for a full minute – and then pant my way through the rest of the class. I found it hard to concentrate on the focus point for the session – sometimes an invitation to investigate the role of the senses, sometimes to meditate on the discipline of *tapas* – the purification of body, speech and mind. I tried not to feel disenchanted when the other students reported tales of meditative ecstasy: 'I felt a tremendous peace. My heart opened up towards the sun. I could feel the *kundalini* energy rising and the crown *chakra* opening up – the thousand-petalled lotus unfurling. It was very blissful'; 'I just feel the breath, I become one with the breath'; 'I meditated on *santosha*, the contentment of being who I am – all of my perfections and imperfections together in one being'.

Sarawathi and Dr Latha Satish would smile encouragingly and the meditation session became known amongst the other students as 'the Bliss Class'.

It seemed ironic that we were trying to find peace of mind in one of the noisiest and most polluted cities in India, if not the world. Chennai might have been steeped in history, home to the ancient Cholas and Pallavan dynasties which died out in the thirteenth century, a settlement for Armenian and Portugese traders, and heavily influenced by the British, having been founded by Sir Francis Day of the East India Company in 1639, but these days it was India at its most intense. There were all the signs of growing wealth I had seen in Pune, Bangalore and

Delhi – coffee shops, endless iWays (a broadband internet chain), vast, air-conditioned cinemas featuring the latest Hollywood plot line along-side escapist Bollywood dreams, Italian, Mexican and Chinese restaurants, Holiday Inn and Sheraton hotels with pools, bars, gyms and spas, glossy designer shops, European interior showrooms – and then there were the all-too-familiar trademarks of urban poverty – open sewers, women and men passed out on the pavement, mangy dogs, and the smell of alcohol on the breath of black-skinned, red-eyed rickshaw drivers. The journey back to the hotel was an exercise in Dragon Man's *aparigraha* – though this time we were talking non-attachment to life itself. Liv, Johan and I would squeeze into the back of the rickshaw and talk over the top of the fear that squeezed our stomachs, trying to ignore the kamikaze tactics of our driver, who grazed the almighty wheels of mighty trucks, squeezed between lanes at traffic lights and ignored red lights completely.

Our hotel, the New Woodlands, had been recommended by KYM and read, on the Internet, as if it was a sweet little vegetarian hotel still lovingly run by its owner. It was, in fact, a small town, comprising a florist, a general store, a travel company and two beauty parlours – one for men and one for women. It was big enough to accommodate a book launch, a celebration of puberty, an engagement party and an Indian wedding running concurrently – and Indian weddings are not small affairs. Every night at least one golden-turbaned groom would arrive on bejewelled horseback and enter the floodlit vivid green garden, with its waterfall and marble statues. Drums, Carnatic singing and the whoops of drunkenly exuberant mates, their arms draped over each other's slim shoulders in a last show of brotherly solidarity, would accompany him. On any given day, horns blared, telephones rang unanswered, the Tannoy from the hotel next door announced an endless stream of taxi arrivals, drivers whose cars played tunes when the key was put in the ignition left it in that position as a substitute for the car stereo they couldn't afford, pneumatic drills reconstructed the swimming pool, lorries unloaded sound equipment, and waiters, in dark beige shirts with brown trousers and Nehru hats, plotted a determined course between bedrooms and kitchen, their expressions ranging from tolerance to open hostility. Tips were inspected in front of your eyes and if found wanting they let you know about it. One waiter took my newspaper and went through my bin, looking to supplement a tip he considered to be on the low side.

Why did I stay there for the whole month – my sleep entirely reliant on earplugs? It wasn't the bedroom – a single bed with a brick for a pillow, a plastic leather-effect chair, brown nylon curtains, speckled brown floor tiles and shabby walls – and it wasn't the shower, which, when it worked, spouted a stream of dark yellow water. It might have been the price – 495 rupees a night – as well as the fact that there were few other options. I looked at the Hotel Shelter but it was so bland that it could have been anywhere in the world, and at the Andrha Mahila Sabha, otherwise known as 'Tourist Hotel'. It advertized itself as 'comfortable stay and vegetarian food'. But despite the promise of 'egg served your style', its iron beds and lumpy mattresses reminded me too much of the Mysore Kaveri Lodge and the pale Dubliner, Sean.

Mainly I stayed at the New Woodlands because we had each other. Johan, Liv, Bruno and I became 'The Gang of Four'. Bruno was not on our course, but he was Johan's next-door neighbour – a very sexy French writer with a mischievous grin, a Francis Bacon screensaver and some interesting anecdotes: 'I 'ad a beer with Noam Chomsky. My teacher love 'eem. 'Eee [Noam Chomsky] always wear the same tie so 'eee don't 'ave to tink about notink.' I wished I could have introduced him to Kedarnarth, the man on the train to Chennai.

Johan, Liv, Bruno and I had planned to spend the first weekend on the beach in Mahabalipuram, an hour's drive south of Chennai. We couldn't wait to get away – we wanted to swim and get some fresh air after being cooped up in a classroom all week. We left Friday's 'Bliss Class' ten minutes early and went back to the hotel to pick up the car that it had taken me an hour to organize the previous day. The car didn't show up and two hours and four phone calls later we decided to abandon our mission and surrender to the apparent will of the universe – we went to soothe our over-stimulated Shakti energy in the five-star Taj Connemara bar. This was a bit of a culture shock after a week in a yoga classroom, especially as there was a TV at one end of the bar showing scantily clad women on a 'Fashion TV' swimwear show, and at the other end two singing Filipino girls. I had a glass of Indian Chenin Blanc. I hadn't had a drink since that other five-star haven, the Ananda in the Himalaya, so within five minutes I was happily singing along to the Filipino girls' covers of Britney Spears and Madonna. The girls, identical twins in matching turquoise spangled tops and tight black satin trousers, looked like Asia's answer to the Cheeky Girls, but they didn't have quite the same level of enthusiasm. Their cover of 'Hotel California' was interrupted by a drunk Western woman (not me) who clambered on stage and gyrated as her two-year-old slept on a bar stool and her husband whooped and hollered.

In between the Britney and Madonna covers we established that Johan was a Leo – 'everybody loves me even though I don't do anything to attract them' – and the rest of us were Virgos. My mind was in the coveted state of *niruddham* up until this point – a veritable 'flawless diamond'; the Boss would have been proud of me. After that it all got a bit hazy. I think that Bruno explained the plot for his first novel, which involved a family, some crazy men with bombs in their heads, an island and a Mexican – at least that's all I could recall of it the next day. At closing time the four of us wobbled off to reception to ask about the possibility of staying in the hotel's presidential suite. The fact that it was $400 a night seemed to present us with no problems – the only real issue was the fact that it had no jacuzzi.

I woke the next day with a bad hangover but felt duty bound to go to Sir's Saturday morning public lecture. Pretty much everyone from school was there. His talks were a heady mix of higher yogic concepts – *samskara*, *samkalpa* and *samyoga* – but in my hungover state all I could do was take copious notes in the hope that they would make more sense to me when I had recovered. I am afraid that I then turned down the chance to do some post-lecture chanting in favour of breakfast with the Gang of Four, and some shopping.

We had breakfast at Amethyst – the café that would become our favourite Saturday morning hangout. We sat on the deep veranda that wrapped itself around the warm yellow *chunam* façade, a house once owned by Jeypore princes, and stuffed ourselves with eggs, sausages and bacon, baked beans, cereal, toast, banana cake, coffee and juice. The courtyard, with its marble tables, wrought-iron furniture and white parasols, was full of Chennai's yuppies, busy making friends and influencing people. Sitting amongst the oasis of greenery, smoking *hookah* pipes flavoured with mango and cinnamon, they talked loudly in English about their latest ads, introducing themselves to each other as 'Akash – he did the launch spots for the Indian State Bank campaign' or Iravan – who apparently was being considered for a creative directorship at BBDO.

Everyone bar Bruno would shop in the glamorous 'lifestyle' boutique next door to the restaurant, which was packed with stylish Indian homeware and designer clothes. I was the biggest Amethyst addict – justifying the purchase of several floaty tops on the 'it's not what you spend it's what you save' logic. Making my way around Chennai had only taught me to relinquish my attachment to life itself; I hadn't quite worked out how to relinquish my attachment to pretty clothes. Eventually we tore ourselves away from Amethyst but only in favour of more shops. We spent the rest of the day hanging out with lots of Indian teenagers in Spencer's Plaza – a huge shopping mall spanning several blocks; young boys held hands as a mark of friendship as they wandered along the airless fluorescent walkways, gathering in the Landmark bookshop to pore over Western copies of *Vogue* and *Elle*, draping themselves over each other as they stared in endless fascination at the scantily clad women breaking every Hindu and Muslim taboo. Liv, Roxanne and I also longed for *Vogue* and *Yoga Journal;* they looked so familiar and reminded us of our lives back home, but they were 500 rupees each and so we joined the Indian girls browsing the bargains in Miss India – 'buy one sari, get one free' – and trying on armfuls of brightly coloured trinkets, which we could wear to the party we'd all been invited to that night.

This first Saturday in Chennai was Valentine's Day. To celebrate, Savannah, the southern blonde mom with peaches and cream skin, had invited us all to meet for drinks in her hotel bar. The Park was only ten minutes up the road from the New Woodlands but it was several decades away in design. Where the Woodlands had the seventies-style marble floors and smoked glass of the Southern Star in Mysore, and exhausted-looking formally dressed reception staff, the Park had men in T-shirts who looked as if they were resting between modelling assignments, curved glass panels, aromatherapy candles and ten didgeridoo-shaped sculptures.

When we arrived the party in the bar was already in full swing. Savannah was perched atop a funky leather cube. 'Hi y'all, welcome to my hotel,' she said. 'I hope y'all feel right at home.' Kausthub was just leaving. His eyes twinkled as he remarked how touching it was to see 'a group of yogis drinking *pranayama* in the Leather Bar'.

Harley distributed chocolate hearts and hugs to the girls and we ordered Ernest Hemingway cocktails. We settled onto our leather cubes to watch Jenifer (representing Illinois) and Annie (Devon) dance to Asian fusion from *Blue Planet–Masala*, which the DJ had picked up on a visit to London. Jenifer and Annie had some serious dance moves – they even persuaded an initially shy Indian girl on a night out with her boyfriend to join in with their hot mix of salsa and belly dancing rhythms. Her boyfriend was supportive until an unrelated Indian man joined the fun – at which point she was whisked away. Liv joined in and quickly became the target of several men's affections, most notably the English cricket A team, who were in need of some escorts to help them get into the hotel's nightclub. Well, we couldn't have left Liv on her own with all those handsome guys, could we? We selflessly devoted the next three hours to helping her out – breathing in a heady mix of star cricketers, cigarettes and aftershave.

By Sunday we were even more in need of some fresh air than we had been on Friday night so we joined an unofficial school trip to Mahabalipuram.

We staggered onto the mini bus that one of the senior students had thoughtfully organized, and crawled out of congested Chennai, nursing our hangovers. The fresh air and the sight of the Coromandel coast and palm trees almost made up for the troubled journey in which the driver got constantly lost, drove single-mindedly over every bump in the road and nearly killed us at least three times.

The Ideal Beach Resort was well named. It had a pool, a poolside bar, a white sandy beach and a shady restaurant serving garden fruit juices, salads and a delicious fish tikka. We all had good intentions – reviewing our class notes, learning our chants and committing to memory the Sanskrit names of the *asanas* we had practised that week – but there were too many distractions for everyone except Beckle, who went to sleep.

Liv played volleyball, her athletic body and Scandinavian good looks bewitching the Lufthansa flight crew on a stopover; Bruno and his shoulder blade to shoulder blade angel wings tattoo frolicked in the waves, and I sucked a little too hard on my coconut juice straw as I watched him. I ventured into the sea, trying to get in touch with Bruno and my inner Ursula Andress, but I ended up getting dumped on by a wave and nearly losing my bikini bottoms. Johan took himself off for massage and meditation and when he came back he shared his hammock with Roxanne, the fun-loving Sydney-sider.

'How many times a week do you polish your pearl?' asked Johan.

'I don't do my own housework,' came the swift reply.

After an end-of-the-day Pina Colada we made our happy, sunkissed way back to Chennai. The Gang of Four took up residence on Johan's balcony, lit some candles, ordered masala dosas and strawberry-pink milkshakes on room service, and listened to thirty-three Radiohead songs on Bruno's computer, drowning out the noise of the Tannoy, taxi tunes and drums below. If we shrank into the back of our plastic chairs we avoided the view of the hotel building and saw only the scraggly tops of palm trees lit up against the black sky. From this angle Chennai looked as sexy as Bruno.

~ 12 ~

'My kleshas really fucked me'

onday morning dawned bright, early and way too soon.

Unsurprisingly the weekend activities had done little to fast-track me to the top of the class. My memory, pickled in Chenin Blanc, Ernest Hemingways and Pina Colada, had been wiped clean of the chants we had learnt last week, and my ability to speak body language had not been improved by close observation of the English cricket A team. My resting state of mind was still that of a ten-year-old, and the *ksiptam* butterflies stirred by thoughts of Bruno and the beach were interrupted by occasional excursions into the *mudham* blues – the thick fog that only Harley and I seemed to be encountering in the Philosophy class.

The usual frustrations were overlaid by a new problem. My neck had started to hurt. At first I put it down to the hotel's brick pillows but it was just as sore after a night on the soft one that I picked up for 50 rupees in one of the town's many pillow and mattress shops (what did they do with all that bedding?). Fortunately I already had an appointment with Dr N. Chandrasekaran, Dr N.C. for short.

The consultation was a necessary precursor to a one-to-one *asana* lesson with my personal yoga teacher – none other than Mekhala herself. She came along to the consultation to watch Dr N.C. conduct his assessment. He was a kind, diminutive man who eschewed *veshtis* in favour of Western dress and wore low-slung, pleated blue trousers, tightly belted under his small potbelly, though he retained the KYM signature pen in shirt pocket. He watched me do some simple stretches, bending forwards and backwards and to the side. I was delighted when he said to Mekhala, 'She is very flexible; did you see her *uttanasana*?' Perhaps all that time spent walking like a horse and stretching my upper eyelashes in Rishikesh had been worth it. He asked me to lie down on the couch and studied me with a critical, well-practised eye: 'Left hip is tighting, and lower back sore.'

'Is it paining?' asked Mekhala. I told her it wasn't but that I had been experiencing some neck pain. Dr N.C. was already one step ahead of me. 'Yes, Lucy, your right shoulder is higher than the left. This must be corrected.' He read my pulses and deemed me, as Vinay P. Menon had, to be *vata* dominant. No progress there then. To counter my impatience he prescribed the chanting of twelve OM *shanties* before bedtime. Apparently I was still a stressed-out Londoner – three months after leaving home. How depressing. When I went to see Mekhala for my private consultation a couple of days later she read my pulse again. Despite the religious chanting of twelve OM *shanties* there was no change – still too much *vata*. She gave me a gentle, repetitious *asana* practice to correct the balance of my shoulders and to build feelings of patience and calm.

I struggled my way through the group *asana* classes – Dr N.C. was teaching at Vedavani this week so he was able to keep an eye on me. I thought I had really slowed down but he kept telling me to relax. By the end of the second week my body felt awful – as if it had decided that if it was only required to do Pensioner's Yoga it might as well become a pensioner – and there was still no improvement in my neck; in fact, it seemed to be getting worse. Savannah had a look at it for me and thought that one of my vertebrae had shifted out of position. In one blissful lunchtime, using a technique called 'acupolarity', involving gentle pressure on two acupressure points, she managed a miracle. There it was, back in place – 'snug as a bug' as she put it. Unfortunately it popped out again the next day, as we were doing some twists in the *asana* class. Ouch. I went running to see Dr N.C, who seemed a bit fraught. I resisted the temptation to suggest he did some OM *shanties*. He took my pulse and sighed.

'Too much *vata*. You must learn how to breathe, Lucy.'

'But Dr N.C., how can breathing move a vertebrae back into position?'

'Lucy, we have cured slipped discs with breathing.'

'How?'

'Because breathing energizes your 72,000 nadis.'

'I see,' I said, not really seeing.

'Do this *pranayama* twice a day and come and see me again next week.'

I left Dr N.C.'s office unconvinced. How could a set of breathing exercises, and a yoga programme that a pensioner would laugh at, sort out my problem?

Not only was my neck not getting any better I was also losing all muscle definition. None of our teachers had the sculpted lean muscles I had been dreaming of; beneath the saris and shirts I detected potbellies and flabby arms. I was grateful that there were no Mysore-style poolside body contests here, but at the same time I didn't want to go home looking as if I had spent six months on bed rest. I knew it was possible for me to build muscle; under the strict guidance of the Swoony Swami my arms and stomach muscles had been strong enough to keep me in *chaturanga dandasana*, the press-up position, for several breaths and, thanks to numerous leg raises, my Cumberland sausage legs had thinned out into chipolatas. Here I was porking up again and I didn't like it.

For some light relief I spent Friday night with the Gang of Four, and half of our class, at a production of *Grease*, held in the Chinmaya Heritage Centre in the north-western suburb of Chetpet. I cheered up at the sight of soft velvet seats and happily settled down to watch the 'we couldn't have done this without you' messages: 'Thanks to the Bounce Style Lounge for hair and styling'; 'Thanks to the fruit shop on Greams Road'; and 'To Menali for bringing us the *Grease* CD from the US'.

We hadn't been quite sure what to expect – *Grease* in saris? In fact it was a completely faithful rendition, right down to the swagger in Danny Zuko's walk and Rizzo's bored disaffection. We sang along and I forgot about the *mudham* blues until the 'Beauty School Dropout' scene. As the white-suited imitator of fifties teen idol Frankie Avalon told Frenchy to go back to school, I had a sinking feeling. This was depressingly familiar. Like Frenchy I was having trouble in class, yet I was surrounded by perfection. There it was before me on the stage, angels in silver dresses and halos, and there they were in the audience, our class fanned out down the rows, dressed in civvies but yoga angels one and all, except Bruno – but then he never set out to be one.

Was I about to become a yoga school dropout? My faith in the KYM yoga dynasty was crumbling. I'd waited a long time for this course, booked it ages ago, I'd loved the theory of KYM teachings, and now that I was here I was impatient for progress. The *asana* classes were too slow, the endless questions took up too much time, I couldn't understand the *sutra* classes – which I'd been really looking forward to studying, I wasn't picking up body language as fast as I would have liked, I was still being whipped by the winds of *vata*, I couldn't open my crown *chakra* in the so-called 'Bliss Class', and we weren't seeing anything of Sir apart from the Saturday morning talks. How was I going to get anywhere? How could I achieve my dream of becoming a serene and poised Yoga Goddess if I had a knackered neck?

Should I move on, find a new school? There were still plenty to choose from. How about the exotic-sounding Danny Paradise (rock star or yoga guru?) at the Purple Valley Yoga Centre in Goa? Or perhaps, if I could get over my hair issues, I should head back up north, to the Bihar School of Yoga. And I definitely wanted to give Auroville a try. Caroline, the reality TV producer I met on that first yoga holiday in Turkey, had spent a month in this utopian community built on the principles of human unity and self-sufficiency – she'd shown me photographs of thirty environmentally friendly windmills over a glass of Pinot Grigio in Julie's Wine Bar. Founded by the Mother, a French disciple of the Bengali yogi Sri Aurobindo, it calls itself a laboratory for the next stage in human evolution, 'a universal township,' as the Mother called it, 'where men and women of all countries are able to live in peace and progressive harmony, above all creeds, all politics and all nationalities.' I was intrigued by the prospect of living in human unity with 1,700 people from thirty-six countries. Ramana Maharshi's ashram was also just up the road. I had wanted to visit the place ever since Jim had shown me a picture of this fine-featured, gentle-looking man with a luminous, peace-conferring gaze.

I put off making a decision with a variety of distractions that whiled away the rest of the weekend. The one that worked best was the trip to Panagal Park – a busy roundabout circled by Chennai's numerous silk shops. Chinnasami Chetty was like an old-fashioned Grace Brothers style department store – attentive staff lifted huge rolls of material from mahogany shelves and laid the fabrics lovingly on their counters. The choice was bewildering so I called on the services of Chitra, who owned a tailoring shop across the street. She was a large woman prone to burping but I felt safe in her hands.

She sailed around the shop, her portly proportions leading the way, ordering the sales assistants to pull out fabrics from the top shelves, pointing out discounts: 'See this, much saving, madam; two thousand rupees to seven hundred and fifty.' An hour later, under her expert guidance, I had enough cloth for four silk chiffon tops and three *salwar kameez* – all for £35. We adjourned to her tiny office where we sipped *chai* as she measured up, a large relative resplendent in a royal purple sari taking up at least half the available space and burping quietly but steadily as she worked her way through a packet of chowgri biscuits. In between her own ever louder burps, Chitra told me that the clothes would be ready three days later; no matter that her mother, in hospital with diabetes-related complications, might have to have her foot amputated. I told her not to worry, that I would understand if there were delays, but she assured me that her word was her bond: 'I am in pain, my mother is in pain, but I am having ten tailors, all are working hard. I am not employing scoundrels. Your clothes will be ready – like the Britisher we are fully on time.'

Sitting on the beach at the Ideal Beach resort the next day, as I watched Bruno frolicking in the waves, I decided to stick around for a few more days. I wasn't optimistic, but at least there were one or two compensations.

I arrived late to the first *sutras* class of the new week. Feeling very Monday morningish, I took up my usual position towards the back of the class, expecting to have to muddle through, relying on the translations in my textbook.

The Boss was talking about '*duhkha*': 'It means distress, suffering, feeling as if you are in a dark room, isn't it. It's the opposite of *sukha*, which means "lightness" – feeling at ease, comfortable in ourselves.' He went on: 'When the space around the solar plexus is constricted it is *duhkha*.' For once I completely understood what the Boss was saying; in fact, it was as if he were in my head.

'The causes of *duhkha* are the five *kleshas* or obstacles ... like a germ deep inside.' These afflictions are responsible for all our sorrows. 'Yoga is trying to remove this suffering' to make it possible for the Eternal Self to see clearly without any of the obstacles getting in the way of a 'mind like a flawless diamond'.

Then he drew the roots of a tree and called them *avidya* or 'mis-apprehension'. 'Ninety-nine per cent of the time we are in the state of *avidya* – it gets in the way of clear understanding but it's not always easy to see – it's easier to see the rest of the tree because it's above ground.' He drew the tree's trunk and named it *asmita* – 'false identity' or 'ego'. The first branch is attachment or *raga* – the desires that we think will bring us happiness but will never go away because what we have is never enough. *Dvesa* means 'hatred', 'unreasonable dislikes' – rejecting people or experiences because they have brought us pain in the past. The third branch is usually the most hidden and can be the most difficult to over-come – *abhinivesa*, which means love of the material and physical life, and all of the anxiety and fear that such attachment can bring. These obstacles could all be active at once, or some could be dormant, and often one branch's activity could wake up another's. The Boss told us that 'everything is not totally independent, everything is intercon-nected'. Suddenly, for a moment at least, my mind was crystal clear, a flawless diamond.

I had been having a major case of *avidya*; labouring under some seri-ous misapprehensions. It dawned on me that the problem was my expectations, not KYM or the teachers. I had set myself all these goals – to return from India fluent in body language, effortlessly performing advanced postures – and yet I was so unaware of what was going on in my body that I hadn't even been conscious of my neck problem, which, when I thought about it, I'd had since Mysore, where I'd spent a lot of time trying to stand on my head. And now, far from supporting me whilst I stood on my head, my neck couldn't even support my head when I was standing on my own two feet. I remembered an anecdote that Kausthub has told us about his grandfather and a student:

'The student came to my grandfather and said, "Sir, I have come to get certified by you that I am the greatest yogi." My grandfather says, "Come tomorrow at six a.m." The following morning he asks his student, "Can you do headstand?" "Yes," says the student, and stands on his head to prove it. "This is not headstand," says my grandfather. "Why are you opening your eyes?" The next day the student goes into headstand again. This time he shuts his eyes but talks. "This is not headstand," says my grandfather. "No good if you are talking." On the third day my grandfather watches his pupil go into headstand and decides to give him some instructions: "Now start breathing slowly. Breathe in and out, for some time." When the student comes out of headstand he asks his teacher, "Why was I finding it so difficult to breathe?" "Aah," says my grandfather, "today you were in headstand."'

Kausthub had used this example to explain that 'the word "*asana*" comes from the root word "to be", to be totally present, to be totally in a particular position, where the senses are not distracting us'.

'Today *asana* has been made into a photograph,' he said. 'There is no difference between this and gymnastics. We see calendars with photographs of someone balancing on a rock in handstand, the sun setting between their hands, yoga in front of waterfalls, even naked yoga. But *asana* is not a performance, *asana* is what happens in the posture and afterwards. A circus man can do many postures – this is not *asana*.' He encouraged us to guard against this by cultivating the qualities of *sthiram* – 'stability, alertness and attention' – and *sukham* – 'remaining light and comfortable in the posture' as we practised. He warned us that *sthiram sukham* should be 'not just in the body – they must be there at the level of the breath and mind also'. This meant no distractions, 'no yoga videos with beautiful sunsets and sunrises on the beach and no TV or music when practising. There must be one hundred per cent *sthiram* and *sukham*,' he said sternly.

Although I hated to admit it, I'd been operating on 1 per cent *sthiram* and *sukham*, and whilst I hadn't been photographed balancing on rocks, it was only because I would have wobbled. Krishnamcharya's student and I seemed to have a lot in common. I needed to start trying to practise *sthiram sukham* at all times; I had to learn 'to be', to be patient, to be here, content with where I found myself, both on and off the mat. And so, several months after my flight landed in Bombay, I began the slow process of truly arriving. As Sir said to us in one of his Saturday morning lectures, 'We begin to open our eyes only when we are in trouble.'

I started by paying more attention to the case studies presented to us by Menaka and her assistant, Shaheeda Murthy. I realized that the impact of KYM's yoga teachings extended way beyond the pupil's *dhurrie*.

We met a highly articulate woman in her thirties who worked full-time for the Southern Railways. She'd begun practising yoga for her diabetes and had found out that she also had high glycerides and high cholesterol: 'I was in shock. As you say "buy one, get one free",' she joked. 'The "eat not" list never ended. I thought it was the end of my happy life. I would have to cook food and not eat it. It was *vairagya*, enforced *vairagya*.' She paused to consider this compulsory renunciation. 'Generally I am a very cheerful person but I became a changed person. I used to see diabetes as something that deprived me of the things that other people have, but now I see that it has been my teacher. I learned to observe myself. Today I was rushing – what was the cause? So through yoga and diabetes I have learnt time management and that every action needs review. I have learnt to be more aware of my actions in every way – in relation to my mother-in-law, the Southern Railways and sugar.'

Menaka and Shaheeda also introduced us to the activities of 'KYM-*mitra*' – meaning 'friends' of KYM – a charitable outreach organization for those who would benefit from yoga but couldn't afford to pay for it. The effect of yoga on these severely challenged people was profound. An epileptic teenager had found his seizures reduced from seven to three a day. We met a cerebral palsy victim who had been rejected by his family because he couldn't use the toilet. The KYM yoga teachers taught him how to use yoga to exercise control and he'd been accepted back into the fold. One autistic twelve-year-old girl had started talking for the first time a year ago. Now here she was, addressing a packed classroom: 'Before I was not able to speak, and now you are listening to me.' What unified this pretty diverse group was their attention to their practice – even when they were 'performing' to forty Westerners. A dozen 'slow learner' eight- to twelve-year-olds showed far more focus and concentration than I ever had as they flowed through a sequence of fourteen or fifteen *asana*. Not a single mistake. The Downs Syndrome children at the Mathru Mandir School had plenty of focus on their mats, and in the kitchen – where I watched them make the cookies and muffins they delivered to Vedavani. (Their recipe for Apple Muffins is in the back of the book.) If I could muster half their attention I would be well on my way to the sublime state of *sthiram sukham*.

We also met one of India's greatest dancers, who came to Sir and Menaka a year ago following chemotherapy for cancer. They 'prescribed' lots of lying twists, *pranayama* and chanting to open her lungs and settle her swollen stomach. The results had been jaw-droppingly successful. She told us, 'When I saw my doctor he said, "Your lungs are beautiful – how can you have had pleural eclusion?" Because of this yoga practice my body is back to the way it was.'

'You must have guts and faith,' Sir informed us. 'If you don't have these things, nothing can cure you.' In fact, faith in the ability of yoga to heal was a common ingredient in all of the cases we saw, albeit some-times a little misplaced. One portly sixty-three-year-old man, a retired tailor, was so round that he couldn't twist his body when lying down. He came in with spondylitis, diabetes, myocardia, bronchitis and constipation, and told us, 'I hope that in a few months' time I will be a teenager.' He was also given dietary advice, which he took with a light heart: 'Once in a while you can break the rules. I don't want to be a *sannyasin*. They say I can eat a little white meat but I am worried about bird flu so I think this means I can eat a little red.' None of these people had the kind of yoga body I had dreamed of, but they were all using yoga to positive effect and that was more than could have been said of me. They had control over their minds, bodies and senses. If they could use yoga to triumph over cancer then surely I could have some faith in its ability to mend my neck?

It became clear, observing these case studies, how important the teacher/student relationship was. At last Saturday's public talk, someone had asked Desikachar, 'What should be the priority of yoga in Western countries?' He had replied: 'Relationship. Relationship between teacher and student, between the person who wants to learn and the person who wants to give … [In the West] information is given but there is no relationship. I hope this doesn't happen in India. Without relationship yoga is like a dead body. Relationship is *prana*.'

Someone else had asked why Sir's book, *The Heart of Yoga*, is dedicated to J. Krishnamurti. Sir told us that Krishnamurti had originally asked Krishamacharya to teach him yoga but his father replied that he was too old and he would send his son. Desikachar arrived on a motorcycle to teach this great man. Krishnamurti was by this time, January 1966, known throughout the world as a great spiritual teacher, probably one of the greatest of the twentieth century, and lived in a very fine colonial-style house, but he remained so humble that he refused to sit until Desikachar had done so, even carefully moving an insect out of his way. At this time Desikachar was a very inexperienced teacher: 'I was bluffing and bluffing. I was telling things that were not real. He never questioned me.' The experience taught Sir how to be a good student.

I decided that a girl could do worse than to use Krishnamurti as her role model. I would become a model student; settle down in class, pay attention, keep my faith in yoga's ability to heal, do my OM *shanties*, practise patience and 'just being', observing the workings of my *kleshas* in this new spirit of informed awareness.

I spent the remainder of the course practising this new attitude, with varying degrees of success. I really enjoyed chanting – not minding when I had to chant solo in rehearsals for the performance in front of Sir.

I knew I wasn't taking anyone to the heavens, to the state of *mudita*, but then neither was my pronunciation sending them to hell. My neck began to improve with the help of Savannah's ministrations, the OM *shanties* and Mekhala's *asana* prescription, which I did every night before bedtime. The Vedavani *asana* classes gathered pace and it became all I could do to stay present and focus on the tasks at hand. I certainly didn't need shots of coffee to convince me I was alive afterwards. There were more dazzling bursts of daylight during the remaining Yoga Philosophy classes, and I learned to appreciate the slow rhythms of the 'Bliss Class'. Miracle of miracles, I began to understand how to put an *asana* sequence together that didn't end in 'a never-ending cycle of agony' – I was finally learning to speak body language.

It wasn't all good news. The *kleshas* continued to assail me on a minute-by-minute basis. I struggled with *raga* on the beach, as the sight of Bruno frolicking in the surf filled me with insatiable desire. I battled with Chitra. Her mother's foot had been saved but my tops were not. When she eventually delivered them they were unwearable – too short and too tight. I managed to avoid a full-blown case of *dvesa* – her mother's illness had obviously put her under a lot of pressure, but I still longed for what might have been. The tentacles of *abhinivesa* held me firmly in their grasp.

I could take comfort in the fact that I was not the only one experiencing problems. We were all having trouble staying present, and by the final week of the course attendance and attention were beginning to flag. Students were skipping some of the afternoon classes to shop for going-home presents or to see the sights they had missed – the Theosophical Society gardens or Krishnamurti's house. Many of those who did make it to class, particularly those in the back half of the classroom, were distracted – exchanging notes and daydreaming. The only person who didn't look as though he was about to fall asleep was Beckle, who miraculously spent the final week wide-awake.

Who could blame us for struggling? We had the five *kleshas* to contend with and I think we may have discovered a sixth previously unknown one. An American student with an exemplary body preferred to conduct his *asana* and meditation classes wearing nothing but his red boxer shorts. Surely this had to be the ultimate obstacle to achieving a mind like a flawless diamond?

Apparently even the senior long-term students, who were sitting in on some of our classes and studying with Kausthaub or Sridharan, were not exempt from the influence of the *kleshas*. It was rumoured that they had fallen victim to *raga* and had been compiling a list of those students they would most like to shag. It was said to be in the oral tradition of the *Vedas* and we were therefore unable to prove its existence. Those of us who had heard about it decided, rather sanctimoniously, I thought afterwards, that we would prefer to starve our *kleshas* than to know whether we were on it.

We soldiered on to the end of the week, fighting the now six *kleshas* and the desire to sleep in class. The Valedictory Function passed off without a hitch, the plastic chairs were out in force again, and Beckle led us in a return match of *'Mayi Medham'* – the *Vedic* chant Sir had performed to bless us at the beginning of the course. Our rendition may not have been perfect but I think we avoided casting anyone into hell. Kausthub's daughter donned a pretty orange and green number in which to crawl across the floor towards her grandfather, and the rest of us wore our latest Amethyst, Fab India and tailor-made creations in which to receive our laminated yellow graduation certificates.

Harley had a Saturday-night party to celebrate the end of term, and David's thirty-ninth birthday. As we'd already seen in the Leather Bar at the Park Hotel, some of the yoga students had smart dance moves: the Birthday Boy, in maroon two-tone trousers, black shirt, leather necklace and perfectly groomed beard, gave a very plausible impression of a *Soul Train* dancer; Liv found many enthusiastic supporters of her low-rise red with yellow flowers drawstring trousers; Roxanne and Savannah gave almost perfect imitations of Uma Thurman dancing with John Travolta in the *Pulp Fiction* Jack Rabbit Slims nightclub; Johan looked on appreciatively; I did my impression of a disco bunny; and our garlanded host dished out chilled Ukranian Honey Vodka.

After I had finished impersonating a rabbit, I settled into conversation with curly-haired Swiss Emil. We hadn't really talked much before but I was curious to hear the full, unexpurgated version of the story that had won him the competition that Sir had run in class for the best example of *kleshas* in action.

'Actually,' said Emil, lowering his head towards me, 'I had a massive attack of *raga* – I was craving for a pizza so badly I rang the home delivery service.' The dialogue, he told me, went something like this:

I'd like to order a home delivery pizza, please.

Pasta, sir?

No, pizza.

Pasta, sir?

NO, PIZZA!

Ah, pizza, sir.

Yes, PIZZA!

What kind of pizza, sir?

Green peppers, mushrooms, sweetcorn.

Sorry, sir, I am not catching you.

GREEN PEPPERS, MUSHROOMS, SWEETCORN.

Ham, cheese, pepperoni, sir?

'By this time I had *dvesa* for this man,' confided Emil. 'I really hated him. But now I had to give him the delivery details.'

My name is Emil.

Movie, sir?

MY NAME IS EMIL!

I sorry, sir, I can't hear you.

'This went on for several more minutes,' Emil concluded. 'I put the phone down, furious. I was convinced that it was never going to arrive, and if it did the order would be wrong. The result was total *avidya*, total misunderstanding from start to finish. And then, of course, the perfect pizza arrived.' He paused to reflect. 'My *kleshas* really fucked me.'

At last, a *klesha*-ridden soulmate? I told him that I had once had a Swiss boyfriend.

'Was he good?' asked Emil.

'Oh yes,' I said, 'very.'

'Would you like to try with another Swiss?' ventured Emil.

'Oh yes,' I said, 'definitely', wondering, as I said it, whether I should have played slightly harder to get.

'The problem with most men,' continued Emil thoughtfully, 'is that they are stimulated to enjoy sex visually rather than through the body. I have done many workshops on this with partners – perhaps you have read *Making Love the Divine Way*?'

I promised to get a copy.

'It is a beautiful thing this Divine Way. I became very emotional – I was crying the first time.'

'And how did your partner feel about this?'

'Oh, she thought it was beautiful,' said Emil. 'Most women love this closeness. You're encouraged to stay with your partner for two years.'

'So no more one-night stands?' I asked.

'No, they are too hurtful.'

Sadly Emil and I didn't have two years or even two hours. He was leaving for Switzerland that night. I watched him twirl the sexiest women in the class around the rooftop dance floor, above the twinkling lights of Chennai, and wondered if I might have been the last one to spot an opportunity.

Oh well, it was time for me to head off, too. I had decided to head for Auroville and was looking for a travelling companion to come with me. Beckle told me it was just 'an adventure playground for artists' and that there was something cultist about it. 'It's not India, it's weird shit,' he pronounced. Something told me Bruno wouldn't be my travelling companion either. He wasn't very keen on yoga full stop, and saw no reason to create an exception for Sri Aurobindo's Integral Yoga, even though it was supposed to prepare the world for the next stage in human evolution – the bringing down of a higher so-called 'Supramental Consciousness' into man so that he can become an expression of the Divine on earth.

Sri Aurobindo had acknowledged that this was likely to be quite a challenge for most people, such a challenge in fact that even Lord Krishna hadn't attempted it. But with this said he retired to his bedroom for twenty-four years to give it a try. I think he rather dumped the Mother in it, leaving her to attempt the collective realization of his vision on her own.

Bruno was emphatic. 'I 'ate ziz man Aurobindo. My friend in college – 'ee do a Ph.D in two years and 'ee smoke a lot of grass but 'ee love Aurobindo and 'ee always talk about Supramental Consciousness. I don't agree with a word 'ee say – because I tink you 'ave to live in zee world and 'ee say you must come and live with me separate and I don't tink it is right. You *must* live in zee world. Now I can't talk to my friend any more – 'ee is lost.'

I finally found my travelling companion in Savannah, who was interested in the drawing down of Supramental Consciousness and the prospect of some good shopping – the Auroville shop in Chennai was great, and she thought the shops in the township itself would probably be even better.

We agreed to meet there in a few days, once I had paid a quick visit to Bhagavan Sri Ramana Maharshi's ashram, just west of Auroville. Although I had certainly given up on the battle to achieve mastery over my body I was still keen to collect any techniques that would help me control the ramblings of my mind. I would follow the path of *Jnana* yoga, the yoga of wisdom, insight and true knowledge, to the gentle-faced Maharshi's ashram in Tiruvannamalai. He was a *Jnani*, established in the state of true knowledge, and he had invented a clever method of Self-inquiry that used the mind to dismantle the mind – it might just do the trick.

~ 13 ~

'Not all nine hundred and ninety-nine holes are plugged at once'

I left Chennai as I had arrived – gasping for breath. I was so glad to get out of its smoggy clutches and onto the south-bound, coconut-palmed Coromandel coastal road, passing the fluttering flags of the Ideal Beach Resort, *keet*-thatched huts scorched by the sun to a burnt-out grey and lines of fishermen wading waist-deep across the inlets – straw baskets resting like girlish summer hats on their backs. I gazed out at fields of sugar cane, watermelon and aubergines, bright green rice paddies, and casuarina, banyan and peanut trees. I gulped down the fresh air, eyes watering in the wind, head hanging like a happy dog out of the ubiquitous Ambassador window, looking at the men combing out glistening white salt from squared-off monochromatic plains. I was free at last, giddy with end-of-term excitement.

As we headed west, inland along the bumpy roads of the Palar

Valley, the insistent horns of lorries and irate rickshaw drivers were gradually replaced by the peaceful whirr of cyclists balancing Tiffin pots on their handlebars and the gentle, straining sounds of red and orange horned buffalo pulling carts piled high with melons and people. A solitary man pressed creases into schoolboys' shirts at a roadside ironing stand, whilst those tiny, dark-skinned, beautifully presented women, the workhorses of India, shook coconuts from palm trees, laid sweet-smelling straw to dry across the caked, baked red roads and carried piles of just-made bricks on their heads.

As the fierce heat and topography asserted themselves, we became dwarfed by the hill ranges that rose on either side of the road and silenced by the temperature that rose a degree for every kilometre we travelled towards the interior. We waited at a railway crossing for what seemed like hours; I traded my Brittania 'Eat Healthy Think Better' biscuits for a spot in the shade of a stall closely guarded by a big-eyed small boy. At Gingee, fifteenth-century twin forts faced each other across sheer cliffs 150 metres high. Like all good pilgrims we submitted to these forces greater than ourselves and kept our heads down until we reached our destination, Tiruvannamalai, one of the holiest towns in Tamil Nadu.

I wasn't quite sure what to expect, except that there would be no *asana* classes. According to David Godman in *Be As You Are, The Teachings of Sri Ramana Maharshi,* the guru 'would usually criticize *Hatha* yoga because of its obsession with the body. It is a fundamental premise of his teachings that spiritual problems can only be solved by controlling the mind, and because of this, he never encouraged the practice of spiritual disciplines which devoted themselves primarily to the well-being of the body.'

However, I wouldn't be taking it easy. *Jnana* yoga has a reputation as the hardest of the yogas; the mind goes on a quest for its origin, to examine its own nature. This is done by asking the question: 'Who am I?' As thoughts come up another question is asked: 'To whom has this thought come?' The obvious answer is 'to me', but who is 'me'? Repetition of the 'Who am I?' question will eventually destroy all other thoughts, and in the end the questions will themselves also die. All that will be left is pure awareness – a direct experience of *sat-chit-ananda*, of existence-consciousness-bliss.

I wasn't sure I was going to be able to reach this mental state in three days but I could already see that the ashram was doing everything it could to help. In fact I was pretty soon awarding it the title of 'Ashram of the Year'. Passing beneath a green arched 'Sri Ramanasramam' sign, I entered a world of elegant simplicity: white-washed walls offset by signature green and terracotta detailing; raked sand walkways; rare, milk-white peacocks fanning their tails on the roof and walls.

Having signed the thick leather-bound visitor's book of Dr Murti, who welcomed me, and adding a British address to the hundreds of Swiss, German, French, American and Canadian home towns, I was shown to a modern block, reached by a footpath that ran alongside a tank busy with mosquitoes and bathing *sadhus*. My room would have been described in the 'Best Ashram Review' as 'small but charmingly rustic' – it had signature green shutters to the front and back, a small wooden desk, an iron bed and a terracotta earthenware pot on a bedside table. On the white-washed wall hung some shelves, a picture of the fair-faced, white-haired Ramana Maharshi gazing down with his customary grace, and a mirror – on which a previous occupant with a sense of humour had stuck a 'Who am I?' label.

Dr Murti had given me a timetable. Nothing was compulsory but there was a pretty continuous cycle of *puja* and chanting in the main hall. I went to have a look. For many years the Maharshi's *samadhi* shrine, at the far end of the hall, had been covered by a simple bamboo structure, but this had been dismantled to make way for imposing polished black granite pillars and acres of marble. I sat down to listen to ten ponytailed, ash-smeared *Brahmin* boys, enrolled on the seven-year programme at the ashram's own chanting school, *Veda* Patasala, working their way through a small part of the *Vedas*. They were not as well behaved as we had been in Shovana's chanting class; yawning and wriggling from side to side, they sang not as one but as individuals and were gently chided by their teachers.

The hall was busy with worshippers, young and old. A tiny girl – similar in size to baby Desikachar – crawled determinedly in her shimmering pink nylon dress and petticoats towards the white marble shrine, continuously pulled back by her father just before she reached the raised platform. A constant procession of more grown-up devotees walked clockwise around the shrine performing *giri pradakshina*, a miniature version of the 14-kilometre circumambulation of the Arunachala hill behind the ashram, which Ramana Maharshi prescribed to his followers as auspicious. The devotees were all walking in the same direction but that was about all they had in common. The bronzed, open-shirted, hairy-chested tourist in Bermuda shorts and bumbag looked as if he had banged his head falling off a passing cruise ship and hadn't quite woken up to where he was. He was followed by a waddling, orange-clad *sadhu*, potbellied and heavy-browed, his forehead further accentuated by the horizontal lines of the *Saivite*. Several Indian ladies glided along, seemingly on wheels, in muted saris; a painfully thin traveller girl in huge trousers and tie-dyed tunic top made slightly less elegant progress; and several rather fierce female residents in white pulled up the rear. Colourful backlit photographs showed the timeless Maharshi, softbodied in his loincloth, carrying his two personal possessions – his water pot and walking stick. He seemed to look down with kindness on his devotees in their varying states of dress and undress.

Vedic chanting completed, a bare-chested *swami* bearing armfuls of orange, pink, yellow and white garlands, and a lot of green leaves, conducted a *puja* at the Maharshi's shrine. He scattered the leaves and petals as he chanted, filling the air with a mixture of flower scent, citronella and incense. After the *Arati* lamp and *tilaka* rituals, involving *kumkum* and sandalwood paste, we moved next door to the Maharshi's mother's shrine – built as an expression of the Maharshi's love for his mother, and for all mothers of the world, and around which the ashram had initially grown.

I was just beginning to settle into some more chanting – this time of Ramana Maharshi's *Tamil Parayana* or 'Recitations', the Indian lady on my left finding my place for me whenever I got lost – when I had my first encounter with the 'Near-Naked *Sadhu*'. He wore nothing but a tiny flesh-coloured loincloth, hardly ample coverage for this 6ft 6in vision of rippling manhood. His expression was wild as his hair, and he ran into the hall with his fingers in his ears, stopping abruptly before the lines of male and female chanters at whom he stared unseeing, before running out again. Nobody batted an eyelid. I saw him later on peering out from behind a column in the accommodation block opposite mine. I'm not normally one to complain about seeing a near-naked man, especially one in such good physical shape, but this *sadhu* was more than a little scary. Thankfully he had disappeared by the time I went to bed, after a Schubert concert attended by what must have been the funkiest-looking audience ever – lilac headbands, dreadlocks, skinny T's and mirrored belts mingled with strawberry-blonde Divine Children and serious Indian men in starchy white *kurta pyjamas* as the Western pianist played *Fantasie* in honour of the Maharshi, who radiated goodwill to all men from an oil painting portraying him on a tiger skin in his trademark loincloth.

By the next morning I had fallen out of love with my 'small but charmingly rustic' bedroom: the fan on full power had done nothing to take the edge off the stifling black heat; the mattress was another 'One-Incher' – as experienced at the Sivananda Ashram – and the 6 a.m. bucket of cold water at the end of the corridor did nothing to soothe my stiff muscles. I joined the early-morning milk offering to the Maharshi at his shrine in a very bad mood, made worse by dribbling most of the sweet, yellow liquid down my white trousers.

My sweet tooth found more satisfaction at breakfast time, as the *iddlies*, of which I had never been very fond, were suddenly transformed into food of the gods by the addition of brown sugar. This, combined with some very hot, strong south Indian coffee, restored my desire to mingle with the rest of the human race.

Intriguing group photographs of ashramites occupied every inch of the dining room walls – a mixture of warrior-like *sadhus*, starchy *veshti'd* Indian dignitaries, Mediterranean smiles and square-jawed, broad-shouldered balding Englishmen, the kind of men you would have expected to see staring down from a photograph of 'The Rotherfield Greys First Eleven, 1949', on proud display in the village green pub.

I chatted to my neighbour, a baker from Boulogne, who, after a hard morning's work making the village's baguettes and pain au chocolat, had devoured a book on the Maharshi in one sitting. He had resolved to visit the ashram and Arunachala, the hill that the Maharshi called his 'guru' and 'the world's spiritual heart centre', which he believed to be an embodiment of Shiva. The Baker of Boulogne told me that from the day the sixteen-year-old Maharshi arrived in 1896 until the day he died, in 1950, he never ventured more than 2 miles from its perimeter.

The Baker of Boulogne also told me that the garlanded painting of the Maharshi hunched over his bowl occupied the place where he had always sat in the dining room – watching to make sure that everyone got an equal amount. Apparently equality had reigned supreme: 'Zee rules of sharing were never broken. Even when 'ee was ill 'ee would refuse to take not even one glass of zee orange juice because zee ashram could not afford for all 'ees two hundred followers to 'ave a glass.'

Like the Baker of Boulogne, the Maharshi worked very hard in the kitchen, reportedly chopping vegetables and preparing samba and chut-ney in the early hours of the morning. Meal preparation became a school for spiritual development, the kitchen staff growing wise under his tute-lage. This culinary spiritual guidance wasn't limited to the kitchen staff. He wrote his mother a recipe for poppadoms, a song that was translated by Professor K. Swaminathan. The black gram flour was 'the ego-self, growing in the five-fold body field', which had to be mixed with the 'holy company' of pirandai-juice 'and mind control, the cumin-seed, the pepper of self-restraint, the salt of non-attachment and asafoetida, the aroma of virtuous inclination'.

I decided to go and see the hillside cave where he had written this poem, the place he had lived, on and off, for seventeen years, many of them in silence.

Ramana Maharshi had left his family for Arunachala after an incident in which he had been gripped by a terrible fear of death, followed by the realization that his true nature could never die as it was simply awareness or consciousness. In this Self-Realized state he had arrived at Arunachala and become so absorbed in this new awareness that he forgot about his body. David Godman writes that 'insects chewed away portions of his legs, his body wasted away because he was rarely conscious enough to eat and his hair and fingernails grew to unmanageable lengths'. Eventually his body returned to normal but he remained in this Self-Realized state of consciousness for the rest of his life – never again seeing himself as separate from other beings. I wondered if Rishikesh's Shri Shri Ma Anandamayee would have landed up in the same state if her followers hadn't rescued her.

I was a bit worried about going it alone, as I had seen Near-Naked *Sadhu* lurking by the back gates, but, as I began the gentle climb, I stepped in with three Indian boys who were going on a sketching expedition. They thought escorting 'aunty' was hilarious; they punched each other and squealed with toothy delight but, after the initial excitement, conversation died out and we settled into a relaxed pace more in keeping with the gentle, easygoing pathways that cut their way through the scrub and brushwood. Every so often we would turn a corner and I would gasp in surprise at an unexpected view of town or temple, much to the amusement of the 'Fun Boy Three' who had been here a million times before. We said hello to a tired but smiley *sadhu* sitting halfway up the path, his back to the hazy views of the town below. He bade us 'have a nice day'.

An hour after we started I turned off down to the Virupaksha cave and the boys carried on up towards a rock on which they would perch to draw the ninth-century Arunachaleswara Temple, its nine carved *gopurams*, or towered gateways – four of them 60 metres high – reaching up towards us from the town below.

The cave, at the bottom of a steep path, was built in the shape of a giant OM or *pranava* – said to vibrate with the original sound of the universe. Although it comprised a total of three rooms it was only the third innermost room that bore any resemblance to a cave; the rest looked like a pretty white-washed house. A welcoming OM sign in green, red and yellow hung over the front door.

It was incredibly hot in the cave room, hot and dark, lit only by a single candle. Eventually my eyes adjusted to the light and I could make out the shapes of no less than twenty Western men. The author of *Men Are From Mars, Women Are From Venus* was right – men do like to hang out in caves. Here they all were, cramped into this tiny space, their eyes focused on the *lingam* containing the ashes of a previous occupant, Saint Virupaksha, over which a single candle flickered. A notice informed us that 'as the time arrived for him to leave his body, he asked his devotees to leave him in the cave and return the next day. When they returned his body had been converted to *vibhuti*.' There was nothing to do but sit down and join the guys.

The sign requesting silence meant nothing to the two Indian couples that bustled in – by the same rule that says Indians' mealtimes are for eating not talking, caves are for talking, not meditating. They stood in the doorway discussing the heat in proud English, and whether the camera would work in the dark. The two large ladies sat down and mopped their brows. Less than three minutes later they struggled, with great difficulty, and much humphing, back onto their feet and left, one declaring, 'Much heat is happening, I cannot be standing it.'

The spell broken I also struggled to my feet, walking quickly past the highly excitable monkeys playing on the pathway, towards the second of the Maharshi's hillside abodes, Skandasramam, higher up on the eastern slope. He had moved here for the sake of his mother, who had come to live with her son in 1916 but hadn't settled in the cave. They lived here, in this house built for the Maharshi by a devotee, until his mother died six years later. Here again were the signature white-washed walls and green shutters, and that old familiar smell of monkey – so strong it took me back to those rain-soaked days in Rishikesh, although Ram Jhula bridge and Swargashram seemed a lifetime ago now.

There were two people already meditating in the cramped darkness of the little house's inner chamber, several more waiting to go in, including an Indian man who had been waiting so long he had fallen asleep and was now snoring very loudly. Not reckoning my chances of a satisfactory meditation session I went to sit outside on one of the benches overlooking the valley below.

I found myself soaking up the sun next to Dave, a painter and decorator from Southend-on-Sea who had been coming to the ashram for fifteen years. He gave me a piece of his sweet rubbery jackfruit, and lots of tales from the ashram. I had spotted an ancient *swami* in dark sunglasses and thin long beard, who looked like a member of ZZ Top. Dave told me that this was Swami Ramananda – Ramana Maharshi's nephew.

'If he wasn't his nephew he would have been chucked out a long time ago,' said Dave. 'My bedroom's really near his and mine is like a prison cell, but his – well, he's got a TV and a fridge and he likes to have "the lads in *lungis*" round.' We laughed. Dave went on. 'Swami Ramananda has three sons: Ganesan lives just up the road from the ashram and gives *satsang* some mornings; Ramanan is the current president of the ashram – you've probably seen him welcoming people outside the dining room; and then there is Mani – who is in danger of being ousted by Dr Murti who runs all the accommodation for visitors and is becoming increasingly powerful. Dr Murti isn't a *Brahmin* – the priest caste, he's the next one down – a *Kshatriyas* – that's the warrior caste. He's good-looking and has a reputation as a bit of a charmer.'

I explained that I had found him charming but all he had given me was a room key. Dave offered me a potential consolation prize, but warned, 'Mani's daughter married a Western man and now the family are trying to avoid their thirty-something son going the same way.'

Now that would be something; would joining the family firm be a fast-track to a merger with cosmic bliss, when all else had failed? Somehow I doubted it, but Dave looked at me with a glimmer of mischief in his eye, 'Go and see Mani,' he said.

I went the next morning.

Mani was in the office, as was his father who was having a sneezing fit. I thought I would check that this old rock star of a man really was who Dave said he was.

'Yes,' said Mani, 'but now he has taken the vows of *sannyas* and he is no longer my father.'

His father sneezed again, three times, violently. I asked Mani if I could visit Ganesan.

Mani was initially protective. 'He leads a reclusive life – not so much activity these days.' Then he softened. 'He lives a kilometre down the road, you can go to his *satsang* today, if you wish.'

I didn't like to mention the possibility of meeting Mani's son and, unsurprisingly, he didn't suggest it.

I took a rickshaw up the road, passing several orange-clad, barefoot *sadhus* clutching Tiffin pots and walking sticks, performing the circumambulation of the hill in the intense heat.

Ganesan's unassuming house was at the end of a long drive and quite cut off from the road, hiding behind a long row of trees. Five or six Westerners and one Indian man were already in position, spread out across three rows of white plastic chairs on the straw-matted veranda. Ganesan lay before us on a sun lounger, his eyes shut behind round, tinted glasses, his chin hidden behind a grey white beard. He'd had a heart bypass not long ago and seemed frail – there was a pillow under his legs and another behind his head, and his slight frame was covered by a blanket – but when he opened his eyes it was clear that he'd lost none of his spirit. He was, like his brothers, handsome in a neat, intelligent, well-groomed way, but whilst his brothers seemed quite serious, Ganesan had a twinkle in his eye and clearly enjoyed the role of raconteur.

He proudly asserted, 'There is no pre-plan, I just come and talk.' It was clearly our role to just sit and listen. 'It doesn't matter what is being said. Listening is being, so just be. Being in silence plugs the holes in the mind. Not all nine hundred and ninety-nine holes are plugged at once. My secretary – in three years she has been working for me – two hundred holes are now plugged.'

He expanded on his theme: 'On the wisdom path patience is more important than the effort. Take a rock. In breaking the rock the first stroke is as important as the twentieth. Only a fool would say it was the twentieth blow that broke it.'

He moved on to the familiar theme of mind control: 'Chant God's name to make the mind merge back into the Self ...When there is no mind the solution comes. You call it a miracle.' He chuckled as if he would call it something else. 'As long as the mind is there, there is the possibility to be robbed.' 'We are a slave to environmental circumstance; we are a slave to the mind. We must shift from mind to Self.'

I wasn't quite sure what to make of his next comment. He pointed to the white stripe and red dot on his forehead and said, 'My friends ask me why I am wearing these marks on my forehead. I have no religiosity, no *puja*, no *japa*. I wear it for myself – it is make-up – not for reaction. Just for the Self.' From the expression on his face it seemed pretty clear that he was having a little joke with us. Thing was, I wasn't quite sure which bit was the joke.

I'd enjoyed the enigmatic statements emanating from behind the tinted glasses on the veranda of the hidden house; it felt like a small glimpse behind the scenes. I wasn't quite sure that much had been revealed but it had been fascinating nonetheless. I shared a rickshaw back to the ashram with a small, bespectacled man. As he put it, 'I am black and you are white and we are together in thinking this is of interest. That was a most thought-provoking morning.'

Lunch came early in the ashram, at eleven-thirty. The diet seemed to be 'Snikta' – all carbs and no protein, except for some buttermilk, like Atkins in reverse.

I sat next to Dave on the floor, eating off a banana leaf, which we had to sprinkle first with water. I wasn't sure if this was devotional or hygienic but I always made sure I gave it a good dousing. The serving *sadhu* came along with a huge tin bucket, turned it dirty side up, threw the contents of his ladle upon it and beamed. I beamed back, practising non-attachment to *saucha*, and told Dave of my plan to spend some time in the meditation hall that morning. Dave warned me not to overdo it and that 'the Maharshi didn't believe in long periods of meditation. He told Paul Brunton, one of his first Western disciples, that meditation is only for novices. He said in his book *A Search in Secret India*, "The Yogi tries to drive his mind towards the goal, as a cowherd drives a bull with a stick, but on this path the seeker coaxes the bull by holding out a handful of grass." The handful of grass is the question "Who am I?" and the quest for your true Self should be conducted all the time, walking around the ashram, as you're drinking a coffee.'

'I know, Dave,' I said, 'I've read his book, but I just think I might get some extra help in the meditation hall; I am a novice *Jnani* after all.'

Dave wished me well and went for another walk up Arunachala.

Ramana Maharshi had given *darshan* in the meditation hall from 1927 to 1949. He preferred to teach in silence, his gaze supposedly enough to awaken a person's dormant spiritual being. Paul Brunton had written:

> One by one, the questions which I have prepared in the train with such meticulous accuracy drop away ... I know only that a steady river of quietness seems to be flowing near me, that a great peace is penetrating the inner reaches of my being, and that my thought-tortured brain is beginning to arrive at some rest ... Does this man, the Maharishee, emanate the perfume of spiritual peace as the flower emanates fragrance from its petals?

The Maharshi would take up his position in the long, simple hall – sitting for hours on a tiger skin spread out across the divan bed, incense sticks burning, the only sound the swish swish of a *punkah* fan unless, coming out of one of his regular trances, he decided to answer the question put to him by a disciple. The hall would be packed with every form of life – from eminent judges to illiterate beggars, from Jackie the dog – who would sit on an orange cloth and stare at him, not eating until the Maharshi ate – to Lakshmi the cow. Lakshmi had the run of the ashram, as she was believed by the Maharshi to be an incarnation of the 'old lady with the greens', a woman who used to feed the young Maharshi when he lived in Virupaksha cave. According to *Sri Maharshi A Short Life Sketch*, 'Almost every day she [the cow] would find some opportunity to meet Sri Maharshi and she pretty well understood what was spoken to her ... She moved with unmistakable dignity and self-possession, and would not be trifled with nor have anything to do with a person who ill-treated her.'

So, in the presence of a Saint who had been dead for more than fifty years, thought a cow was an incarnation of an old lady and wrote enlightening songs about poppadoms, I sat down to ask myself, 'Who am I?'

I established I was not the tickle in my throat that I had noticed as soon as I was required to be silent. I was not the first grey hair I had noticed in the 'Who am I?' mirror that morning – because soon there would be more of them, and before today there were none of them. I was not the age I am now, because in a second I would be older, and a second ago I was younger. I couldn't be my body because, according to medical research, it had been completely renewed in the last seven years, and, if all went according to plan, it would be renewed again in the next seven.

So, if I was not any of these things then who was I? Perhaps I was my thoughts? My hopes? But my hopes changed all the time, too. Let's take men; in just six months there had been Richard of the full swimming trunks, then Bill and his hammock, then a Swoony Swami, then, fleetingly, Charlie, a mad numerologist from Barcelona and an Italian waiter, then there had been a gap – filled by Divine friendships with MP and Mr Hospitality, the Divine Lifer. Then there was the unrequited lust I had for Bruno and finally there was Mr Divine Love himself, Emil. Many of these hopes, that had filled me with such longing at the time, however fleetingly, were now not only dead, but also looking pretty misguided. Perhaps a nice football-loving English bloke who thought 'The *Kleshas*' were a seventies punk band would be more the thing. Perhaps not. I wasn't quite sure what kind of man I wanted any more but I did know that what I thought I wanted I didn't need.

Perhaps I was my fears? No, these had changed, too. Thanks to the Swoony Swami, Astrid and Cartier, I didn't worry about climbing or descending from mountains any more, and I had come to terms with *iddlies* – as long as they were covered in brown sugar. I was no longer so afraid of travelling on my own that I would pay top dollar to insulate myself against the real India, and I realized that I had actually enjoyed the cheap places most: the Sivananda Ashram had been 700 rupees a night, including all meals, evening entertainment, lectures and yoga; Ramana Maharshi's ashram, my self-appointed winner of 'Ashram of the Year', was free of charge – 'by donation only'.

It dawned on me that if my hopes and fears and body were constantly changing then so was the world around me. Nothing stays the same, not even for a minute except – and this was the essence of Ramana Maharshi's teaching, and in fact of all yoga – the Eternal Self or *purusha*, which remains eternally still.

And then I began to drop; dropping like Jacques Mayol, the dreamily absent freediver immortalized in the film *The Big Blue*, leaving my *kleshas* bobbing around on the choppy water, leaving the flotsam and jetsam of my hopes and fears behind, leaving insistent voices beyond the watery barrier. Sinking deeper into the infinite blackness, becoming very quiet. Sitting on the ocean bed, listening to my breath – deep and steady, watching the air bubbles rising like a thousand reversing raindrops, nothing to worry about, just being, just peace. As Jacques says in the film, 'You go down to the bottom of the sea where the water isn't even blue any more, where the sky's only a memory, and you float there, in the silence.' And there it was, in that weightless inkiness; a stillness, *santosha* or contentment, an awareness of a bigger reality, a place without ego, hatred, cravings, uncertainty and misapprehension. Just pure existence, consciousness, and yes, bliss …

BANG!

I opened my eyes; the door to the meditation hall had slammed shut behind an officious-looking cleaner, who had clearly decided that this was her time for a personal *darshan* with the Maharshi. I wanted to jump up and shout – first at her, for forcing me to come up from the bottom of the ocean so fast I nearly got the bends, and secondly to proclaim to the world that I had just glimpsed *sat-chit-ananda*. It was like riding a bike without stabilisers for the first time – 'Look at me! MUM! DAD! Did you see what I just did?' Feeling dazed, I joined the others leaving the hall.

It was funny that I hadn't been sitting on a mountaintop, as I had always imagined I would be if I ever reached this state, but at the other end of the earth – sitting on the ocean bed. And wasn't it funny that, in that moment of sitting alone on the ocean bed, the feeling of being separate to other people had left me, replaced by a feeling of deep connection

– that I was one of Ramakrishna's droplets of water that jumped into the ocean and said, 'I am That.' Funny that, weird, and probably a bit mad.

As I surfaced, so too did my doubts. Was that really *Jnana* yoga? I had been conscious of my breathing and that wasn't supposed to happen with *Jnana*. The Maharshi hadn't been with me; he hadn't given me 'a thread of silver light' as he had Paul Brunton. How much time had really elapsed? I had experienced a sense of timelessness but when I looked at my watch, no more than a few minutes had gone by. Oh well. Who cared? Whatever it was called, and however long it had lasted, I had felt the potential of a merger with cosmic bliss – without alcohol, spliffs or sunsets – with a man who certainly didn't want to test my blood for HIV before I shared in his energy field, who didn't do hugs, who didn't charge a single rupee in registration fees and who had been dead a very long time.

~ 14 ~

'That's one big-ass crystal'

I left early the next morning, the Ambassador sweeping past several *sadhus* on their third or fourth cup of coffee, reading the paper and smoking *beedis*. There was also an orange-robed man in the Internet café opposite the ashram; was he checking his Hotmail account, or worse? Graham, my lawyer turned yoga teacher friend, had been in Dharamshala seeking an audience with His Holiness the Dalai Lama, and had seen a monk surfing an on-line dating agency. Robe2robe.com?

I was very sorry to be leaving my 'Ashram of the Year' but I had to go. I was meeting Savannah in Pondicherry, at the Sri Aurobindo Ashram. Unfortunately she had to fly home late tonight so we wouldn't be spending much time together, but a day would be enough time to see the ashram and zip the three miles up the road to worship in Auroville's temples – the craft and clothes shops, and at the Matrimandir, literally 'Temple of the Mother'.

I was glad to see photographs of Ramana Maharshi, Sri Aurobindo and the Mother on the Ambassador dashboard. I hoped that they, alongside a golden glittering Ganesh, would offer us some protection on the road. We clocked up four near misses in two hours (versus only three in eight hours when I was in the comparatively safe hands of Ekavir, doing the Delhi to Rishikesh run): one buffalo pulling a haystack; one goatherd; one cream bus with go-faster red stripes living up to its 'Express' name; and one Tiffin-laden cyclist. Ali, the driver, apparently deemed them ready to meet their maker. Having nearly crashed into the back of the bus, he swerved and overtook on a blind corner, laughing like a maniac.

'Why are you all such crazy drivers?' I asked, my knuckles white with fear.

He didn't seem to have detected the note of criticism in my voice. 'Yes, yes,' he laughed. 'Crazy. Totally crazy.'

I tried to remind myself that the path between 'Ashram of the Year' and Sri Aurobindo's ashram was well-trodden, and there had been few, if any, deaths. Aurobindo used to send seekers to Tiruvannamalai, and sometimes they came in the opposite direction. Henri Cartier-Bresson, the famous French photographer, had spent time in both ashrams – spookily enough he was there around the time of each sage's death. When Ramana Maharshi died on 14 April 1950 Cartier Bresson reported seeing a shooting star disappearing behind Arunachala at 8.47 p.m. – the exact moment of the Maharshi's last breath – and he'd taken the last pictures of a ghostly-looking Sri Aurobindo on 24 November in the same year, two weeks before he died.

Miraculously we survived the trip and made our way up through old Pondicherry, a French colony handed back to the Indian government in 1954 but still bearing the French legacy of graceful courtyards and imposing colonial houses behind wrought-iron gates. Savannah was standing outside the ashram entrance on Rue de la Marine. Being a cross between Dolly Parton and Marilyn Monroe, she was surrounded by Indian men. Most were just staring at this tiny bundle of big-boobed, blonde-haired loveliness, but some had managed to maintain their dignity and were busy trying to sell her, with a degree of success, a variety of handbags and bangles. Being a polite southern belle she was not very good at saying no and so the crowds of hawkers grew in line with the number of bags and bangles on her arms. 'Thank you *so* much,' she was saying as I reached her, 'I am *so* grateful to y'all. Y'all are *so* kind, that is *so* beautiful.' She placed another bag on her wrist and payed with a fistful of rupees, clearly way over the odds, judging by the seller's ecstatic face.

For once glad to leave the men behind, we passed through the richly polished wooden gates of the Sri Aurobindo Ashram and into a court-yard that made Kew Gardens look like a desert wasteland. There were flowers everywhere, tumbling over the walls, pushing impatiently out of the ground, hanging from baskets and in every colour of happiness – pink, orange, red, yellow. We followed a small footpath through to a second courtyard in which the marble shrines of Aurobindo and the Mother lay beneath the shade of a huge ancient tree – a Gulmohar, called the 'Happiness Tree' by the Mother.

We joined the varied procession of rich and poor, young and old, pregnant and infirm, families and widows, uniting in silence as we progressed slowly towards the shrines. We knelt down before them, and placed our hands on the heart-shaped bed of red roses, careful to avoid the hundreds of ecstatic humming bees, which were about to faint with happiness. We followed the others in touching our foreheads to the marble surround, a welcome ice pack on a very hot day. The atmosphere was peaceful and devoted, earnest worshippers in utter silence, some sobbing, some smiling and some just sitting. We sat in the peace of the soft grey and white courtyard and looking up at the shuttered wooden porch windows; it was easy to imagine the tiny figure of the Mother appearing on the third-floor balcony to give *darshan* to her devotees down below.

I watched as several people hugged the Happiness Tree. The ashram gardener told me that the Mother believed flowers and trees could channel Supramental Consciousness and that people should use them to express their feelings. She renamed all trees and flowers so that their qualities could be better understood. Sunflowers, of which there were many in the courtyard, were renamed 'Devotion', the Hibiscus was deemed to offer 'Power', and Bougainvillea gave 'Protection' – explaining why it climbed over the wall of the ashram and lined the sides of the roads of Auroville in such abundance.

We moved inside to Sri Aurobindo and the Mother's sitting room – a long thin room dominated by a gold damask and mahogany sofa and two gracious chairs. The previous occupants' pictures smiled down from above the furniture. The Mother reminded me of my Great-aunt Gertrude, who was always as old as the hills, bedridden in a nursing home in the Midlands. I used to be dragged into her dark bedroom and made to kiss this crinkly, skinny old lady who smelled of lavender and pee, her hair slicked back into a bun, her face a mass of sagging folds. The Mother wore a slash of lipstick like a tear across her pale face and fixed me with her beady eyes, but like Great-aunt Gertrude, the red lipstick could not disguise her kind smile, and her head tilted forwards slightly as if she were really concentrating on what you were saying.

Sri Aurobindo had a long nose that gave him a haughty expression, a long white beard that could have been spun by silk worms, and his faraway eyes were unreachable, dreamlike. He might have been a relative of Osho – he also looked ancient, timeless, another intergalactic *Star Wars* hero – but he was so ethereal that he made Osho, with his Gucci goggles and eighties robes, look quite worldly.

As we moved back onto the streets of Pondicherry we discovered that the ashram's influence extended well beyond its own walls. Its soft grey and white signature colours reached into several of the streets beyond, stamping its mark on shops, guesthouses and workshops. Despite the bustle of rickshaws and street traders, these cobbled streets, named after French kings, were quieter and cleaner than the rest of Pondicherry, filled with trees and white-robed folk. We followed the simple grid lines down to the imposing, white-fronted buildings of the seafront, which was separated from the sea by a palm-lined road, resembling the Croisette. As Savannah's entourage grew again it was easy to imagine us in Cannes – a starlet and me, her personal assistant, trying to protect her from unwanted attentions. Eventually, after several stops for photographs with groups of increasingly overexcited Indian men, even Savannah's patience ran out. We jumped into her driver's car and headed north towards Auroville.

I had been expecting Auroville to be an extension of the ashram – containing more white-robed people and cobbled streets with French names, but with the addition of the windmills that Caroline had shown me pictures of.

Well, there were lots of windmills but there were no cobbles and no robes, white, orange or maroon. Instead the Ambassador chased big motorbikes down unsigned dusty red roads, motorbikes driven by men wearing nothing but a pair of jeans. Some of the drivers were a bit wizened, their thin hair tied back in limp ponytails, but many were very very handsome, making me squeal in excitement. There were also girls on big bikes – tiny girls wearing T-shirt dresses and determined expressions, glamorous in their Aviator shades. The Indian people seemed to have smaller bikes on the whole, which they overloaded, as was their custom, with their partner and two children – if married – and if not married, then with entire banana trees, or several of their closest friends.

In view of Savannah's tight schedule we made straight for the Matrimandir. It seemed the logical place to start as it was regarded by the Mother as 'the soul of Auroville', a place 'for trying to find one's consciousness'. Saturday afternoon turned out to be the peak time for finding one's consciousness – huge coaches created a traffic jam to get into the car park, giving up their cargo of hot Indian families with a big sigh of relief.

We stood together in the hundreds-long queue, fanning ourselves with our tiny tickets, losing the battle to stay cool in the ferocious heat. At least Savannah and I were only wearing skirts and loose T-shirts; pity the poor Indian ladies, all of whom were swathed in 6 metres of sari fabric and many of whom carried several additional plump layers. The only consolation was that the queue snaked through some very pretty gardens filled with pink and orange bougainvillea and frangipani – according to the guide book the Mother thought these gardens were 'as important as the *Matrimandir* itself' – a place 'to move from consciousness to consciousness … in the Garden of Youth, they will know youth; in the Garden of Perfection they will know perfection.'

Finally, having perfected our consciousness, and got back in touch with our lost youth, we were face to face with the Matrimandir. From the outside it resembled a giant's golden golf ball, set on a bed of lotus petals, as if it were a trophy on display – each of the 1,400 gold leaf discs glistening proudly against the big blue sky. The ball was slightly squashed, being 30 metres high and 40 metres wide, and enormous golden discs lay scattered on the ground, as if the giant had played a little too enthusiastically, not knowing the power of his swing.

Getting into the Matrimandir was a tough business. Our tickets listed the Mother's many rules for visiting. There would be 'a fixed time or a fixed day to show people around' and was 'only for those who are serious – serious, sincere – who really want to learn to concentrate'. Unlike Osho's place there would be 'no fixed meditations … but they must stay there in silence, in silence and concentration'.

It reminded me of the time the advertising agency had visited Whitehall to discuss the results of our Tobacco Education campaign with a government minister. There were rules, passes, signatures, guards, strict timetables and no personal belongings allowed. Actually Whitehall was more relaxed – even in the post 'Shoe Bomber' days it didn't require you to relinquish your shoes. I felt sorry for the Matrimandir guard, who sat stalwart in the hot sun, facing hundreds of pairs of shoes in neat lines and surrounded by the visitors' surrendered water bottles, cameras and handbags.

I had imagined that once we were inside the giant squashed golf ball we would step into a tranquil golden oasis, but it was a building site. We followed spiralling scaffolding ever upwards, pausing every couple of minutes to let the overheated Indian ladies in front of us catch their breath. Plastic sheeting hung like giant shower curtains from the rafters, deadening the rays of late-afternoon sunshine trying to penetrate the dusty gloom. Were busy weekends seen by Auroville's governing body as a great time to do essential engineering work, just as the British railway authorities did? Nope. Construction work had begun in 1971 and it was still nowhere near finished. I asked the foreman how long he thought it might take to complete.

'I cannot say, it might be one month,' he said. I must have looked doubtful. He tried again. 'It may be one year, or two years, or five years. It depends on many things.'

Mainly it depended on money – around 12 lakh rupees (£14,250) a month, according to one local; she thought the whole thing was a complete waste of money, preferring to meditate under the nearby ancient Banyan tree.

When we finally reached the top of the scaffolding we were allowed precisely one second to take in the sight of the inner chamber – the room Aurovilians use for concentration and drawing down Supramental Consciousness. I had an impression of a spotless round marble chamber bathed in a peaceful half-light and at the centre of the room, on a golden geometric stand, lit from above, a huge transparent crystal globe. As Savannah put it when we got outside, 'That's one big-ass crystal.'

The 'big-ass crystal' didn't please everyone. The Indian visitors were complaining on the way out. No matter to them that it was the biggest crystal in the world, imported from Germany and measuring

70 centimetres in diameter. Where was the *puja*? The incense? The flower garlands? The *kumkum* and sandalwood paste? Where were the potbellied priests with their brass pots of sticky sweet *prasad*? Where were the chanting, restless *Brahmin* boys? Where was the 'Minnie Mouse walking on hot coals' soundtrack? Where was the pink tinsel, the gold streamers? Where were the crawling babies eager to make their way to the shrine?

Personally I would have liked more time with the big-ass crystal, to come back when there were fewer crowds. Aurovilians and visitors staying in the guesthouses were allowed to come early in the morning and late in the afternoon, without the interruption of day-trippers, to better apply themselves to drawing down Supramental Consciousness. Caroline said that she hadn't managed it in the month she was here but she still recommended giving it a go. I had decided to visit Goa and Danny Paradise, but could manage a week.

Meanwhile there was shopping to be done. Savannah didn't have much time to devote to the drawing down of Supramental Consciousness; she had to buy presents for the folks back home. We went to the Visitors' Centre shop where she found plenty of Aurovilian produce to fill the empty suitcase she'd brought especially for this purpose: Maroma's 'Yoga', 'Happy Heart', 'Joy' and 'Inner Peace' aromatherapy shower gels and shampoos for her friends; a hammock for her husband; a wooden boat for her son; a lilac T-shirt and pink trousers for her daughter; linen drawstring trousers and a floaty white top for herself.

After a delicious Provençal vegetable salad in the Visitors' Centre café courtyard – quite the antidote to the 'Snikta' diet of the Sri Ramanasramam – Savannah dropped me at the Afsanah Guesthouse, one of Auroville's oldest guesthouses, near the north-west village of Kottakarai, and left for Chennai airport in a trail of red dust. I was sorry to see her go, but probably not as sorry as the men of Tamil Nadu.

Afsanah, a diminutive, bright-eyed, olive-skinned woman in her mid-fifties, welcomed me, garden shears in one hand, a bunch of flowers in the other. The flowers were destined for the vase next to a large photograph of her father without whose help, she told me, the guesthouse would not have been built. I had been hoping to stay in the room the Dalai Lama had when he came to lay the foundation stone for the Pavilion of Tibetan Culture in 1993, but unfortunately it was fully booked – unsurprisingly it was their most popular room. I ended up in Mirani Cottage, which had a terrace that reminded me of the yoga *shala* at Huzur Vadisi in Turkey – covered in vines, surrounded by long grasses, mynah birds and trees. I lay in my hammock and watched the fairy lights and beacons illuminating the bushes surrounding the Japanese water gardens as the large frog that had been turfed out of the hammock watched me, and the cat sitting on the day bed watched the frog.

That night I slept the sleep of a child; my mattress was several inches thick and the trees surrounding the cottage kept it cool. In the morning I had a proper shower with hot water and soap. The only downside was sharing the circular bathroom, tucked away at the bottom of my garden, with several white frogs – there was one on the tap, which gave me quite a shock when I tried to turn on the shower, but perhaps not as big as the shock I gave her – or her babies, who were sleeping in my towel.

Despite the comforts of Marani cottage my neck had not been helped by the nights spent on the inch-thick mattress at the Sri Ramanasramam, so I arranged a treatment with Henri, apparently the best masseur in the township. I set off on my newly acquired moped for his house in Aurodam, a community very close to the Matrimandir. As was customary in Auroville there were no signs; apparently they got nicked as soon as they were put up. I finally found Henri, after two wrong turns, in a clearing at the end of several forked paths.

He had obviously lived here for a long time; his house was surrounded by a large collection of tatty hosepipes, bashed-up buckets and pushbikes. Opposite his front door was a small temple – an old buffalo skull took the place of the 'big-ass crystal'. To the east was a makeshift artist's studio, a faded painting of a large cuddly bear on its door. The earthy house had somehow become a part of the enchanted wood in which it sat; trees tangled above it and long grass surrounded it. Through the open front door I could see a pile of fruit and vegetables on the kitchen worktop and glimpses of a happy domestic life – cushions and papers, candles and books.

And there was Henri, a heroic, muscular body in old-fashioned shorts, his eyes closed, his lined face raised to the early-morning sunshine, wearing a blissful smile. I took a seat next to him in his 'waiting room' – a stone table under a canopy of green. No magazines – just a collection of shadows waving their way across the table. No music or radio playing in the background – just the sound of the wind in the creaking trees and mynah birds having a chat. After about ten minutes Henri opened his eyes and blinked, releasing huge tears down his cheeks. He smiled through the wetness. 'Hello.'

'Hello,' I replied. 'Were you meditating?'

'Meditating always. It's so beautiful, don't you think? OM.'

I agreed stiffly, wishing that I had the kind of floppy limbs and manner that would have come with being raised in a caravan by hippy parents. 'I'm Lucy,' I said, wishing that my name were Celestine or Iona or Skye, or all three.

'Hello Lucy. Welcome. The temple awaits your body,' he said, directing me towards a tripod construction of casuarina poles, bamboo, coconut rope and *keet*, hidden by the trees. I stripped down to my underwear and he began. As he moved his questioning hands gently over me he asked, 'Is your body giving you pain? OM. What is your body telling you? OM.'

Henri had the air of a boxer, but in the graceful style of Mohammed Ali; his body may have been strong and stocky and his face determined, but he leapt from one side of my body to the other with nimble feet, his

body seemingly weightless. He explored every inch of my spine, pausing every couple of vertebrae to listen to it, and to the wind chimes. 'The
wind is happy today,' he said, with a big smile. Finally he gave his diagnosis: 'Your vertebrae are fusing together because the muscles are
contracting them after years of tension, pulling them tight, tight, tight.
And now you feel nothing in your spine because your body has forgotten how to feel. We must persuade the muscles that it's OK. No fear.
They can let go. Nothing will happen. OM.'

I told him about my experience in Chennai, and how I had only just
realized that I hadn't been practising yoga with attention.

He told me not to worry. 'You will move back into your body,
become aware again, your mind and your body will move together. Yoga
is good when you have body awareness but if the awareness is not there
you can damage yourself. I have seen eighteen yoga teachers in the last
few years – some of them came to me with crippled bodies. So many
injuries are happening.'

He gave me some simple 'Somatics' exercises to do every morning:
these were developed by Thomas Hanna, a disciple of Feldenkrais, a
scientist who knew Einstein and worked in the same area, on movement
and matter. 'He worked out how to bring consciousness back to the
body,' Henri said. 'When you do these exercises it will help you to practise your yoga in a mindful way – you can listen to what your body is
telling you. Do them now.' He watched me perform the five exercises.
'Focus your attention on how you feel inside. Atcha! OM. Relax on your
back and feel the changes. OM. Now show me.' I showed him. 'Beauty.
OM.' I showed him again. He looked at my body as if it was the seventh
wonder of the world. 'Atcha! OM. I am jealous. Your spine would not do
this for me. Now it is playing with me. Beauty. Atcha! OM.'

As he worked I asked Henri how he came to Auroville. 'Actually I
came to India before Auroville was here. I came in nineteen sixty-six to
the [Sri Aurobindo] ashram; I was twenty-four. I took a sea passage from
France to India – I knew I wanted to experience something different, a

new way of living. I thought maybe I'd go to Tibet or Nepal but on the eleven-day passage I had lots of time to read Sri Aurobindo's book *The Life Divine*. OM. I came to Pondicherry, to the ashram. I had no money, just a ticket home; I thought I would stay for forty-one days. I asked to meet the Mother and I was given an appointment for the day before I was due to leave for France.' He paused and looked up at the picture of her that gazed down on the mattress. There were those beady eyes and that kind smile. He went on to describe a feeling just like the one Swami Vijayananda had described when he met Shri Shri Ma Anandamayee: 'The moment that I looked into her eyes I knew. Boom! Life was wide open, vast, expansive. OM.'

'I asked if I could stay and at first she played with me, but then, of course, she said yes. I had been at the ashram for two years and then, on the twenty-eighth of February nineteen sixty-eight the Mother gave birth to Auroville. There was an opening ceremony at the amphitheatre and children came from all over the world to fill an urn with earth from their country. The Mother had been given a map of the land. She closed her eyes and pointed to a spot: "Here is the centre of Auroville – build from here." This spot was where the Banyan tree sat – the only tree for miles around.'

This tree had a lucky escape. The gardener at the Sri Aurobindo Ashram had told me that the tree 'came to the Mother in a vision and asked her if it could stay as it wanted to be part of Auroville – so she gave instructions for it not to be cut down' and the Matrimandir was moved 100 metres to the north.

'At that time there was nothing, just sand,' continued Henri. 'We used to call it "The Red Hills". From the Matrimandir to the sea was one vast expanse of nothing. Nothing.' I couldn't believe that this enchanted wood had not existed forty years ago but Henri was adamant. 'When we first started there wasn't even any water. We used a water diviner from the Tamil village. He would point and we would dig; he was very strict. One time he said, "Dig here" but it suited the

Aurovilians to dig somewhere a little to the left. They dug for thirty metres and hit a big rock. No water. They had to start again, where he had told them to dig.'

Although she'd 'left her body' in 1973, Henri was sure that the Mother had watched over the whole process. 'The Mother is here now. She said, "I invite you to come on this big adventure. I don't know where it is going or what will happen tomorrow – we cannot plan how it will be. It takes shape as we learn, as we experiment."' He paused to reflect, his eyes filling once again with water. 'Life here *is* a big adventure; we are trying to live in a new way with the earth, to do things differently. I feel that I am living a fairy tale but the beauty of the fairy tale is that it is real. Every moment is beautiful. OM.'

At the end of the massage we went into the house. Henri wanted to show me some photographs of Auroville that were taken in 1974. It still looked barren, but there were nascent signs of life – a line of trees to one side and some tripod structures like the massage temple. Henri told me they are called 'capsules'. There were also some people in these photos – lean, muscular men who had put down their tools for a moment to pose for the camera, wearing the big smiles of pioneering heroes, whilst pretty girls with long hair and long skirts looking on admiringly in the background.

'The work was very very hard, very physical. In the beginning I did not do massage but I saw so much need I had to do it. Everybody was in so much tension – not just from the work but also from the fight with the ashram. They would come to the "Aspiration" kitchen and there would be so much "oof".' Henri mimicked someone with shoulders to their ears and a set jaw. 'The fight with the ashram was very serious – when the Mother left her body many ashram people wanted to control Auroville, to turn Auroville into a religious business, but we did not want this. It went all the way to the High Court in Delhi. It got very nasty – Tamil villagers were hired as *goondas* to scare us. In the end it was settled and we were able to move on, but the massage was a way of removing the people's tension. My teacher said, "When you massage forget the separation between your hands and the body. Allow the Mother to come through your touch."'

I didn't really want to leave the fairy tale cottage in the enchanted wood but I had already taken up a lot of Henri's time, my neck was much better, and a Tamil villager was waiting outside with a painfully swollen ankle. I asked Henri how much he charged for a two and a half hour massage. 'You decide, that is if you want to pay,' he said. I pulled out a wad of rupees. He pulled out a book with a photograph of the Mother between its pages. 'Give it to Her. It is for Her that I do this work.' As I left, Henri was speaking in fluent Tamil to the villager.

I spent the week exploring the red lanes, imagining myself as Marianne Faithful in *Girl on a Motorcycle*, on my 50cc scooter. After a couple of days I managed to overtake a granny on a bicycle. I covered all four corners of 'the Galaxy', the architectural principle for the township radiating out from the Matrimandir. From this spiritual centrepoint spun four zones – Cultural, International, Industrial and Residential – but I loved the surrounding Green Belt best. It was here I felt closest to Henri's fairy tale – getting lost in the enchanted woods as flowers nodded in response to the breeze stirred by my 50cc scooter. Auroville's big adventure felt most alive here. In these parts, hidden from the path, easygoing men with wild hair and *tundus* (wide headbands) worked hard, in Henri's words, 'to live in a new way with the earth' – growing organic carrots, papaya, tamarinds, radish, sweet potatoes and passion fruit at Discipline farm, fermenting cow dung as an alternative source of energy and irrigating the burgeoning forest. There were houses here, too, as much a part of the forest as Henri's cottage, made of natural materials, with smooth lines and off-centre windows. Their inhabitants were leathery old ladies in smock dresses, with wild body hair and long boobs untamed by bras, who would suddenly appear on the veranda to watch you pass by.

Auroville's architecture was just as much a part of 'the big adventure' as the people themselves. The Mother had appointed Roger Anger, a form-loving Le Corbusier-inspired French architect, to oversee the physical development of the township, and said that 'Auroville wants to be a field of constant research for architectural expressions, manifesting a new spirit through new forms'. Not all of the early experiments were successful – a bamboo globe built on the edge of the canyon was blown away by the first gust of wind. But there were some notable triumphs – I saw a house in Ami that looked like a Dali-esque meltdown, even more surreal than most of Dali's paintings in its place amongst the cashew fields. This sloping show-off was a contrast to the ironic, angular lines of Savitri Bhavan – a place dedicated to the study of Sri Aurobindo's poem '*Savitri*' – or to the very private Atitha Griha, the terracotta guesthouse tucked away behind the Indian National Pavilion – in which earthen verandas gathered around a Neem tree for moments of quiet introspection.

Eating in Auroville was very much part of the fairy tale. After several months of almost unrelenting Indian food, I felt like Hansel and Gretel when they discovered the Gingerbread House. I was practically breaking off the sugary windows and licking the cakey roof of the township's many restaurants. The majority of Auroville's Western settlers, especially in the early formative years, were French. This meant Gorgonzola cheese, real coffee and homemade quiche on the restaurant menus, and a boulangerie selling pastries, baguettes and pain au chocolat. Pour Tous was quite literally the world's best supermarket, the ingredients supplied by a soil rich in organic goodness, grown under a sun unafraid of its own strength, cooked to French recipes and run by Indians – the world's best shopkeepers.

My early days in Auroville weren't all food and frolicking in the Green Belt. I was, of course, also working on my spiritual development. I am afraid that this wasn't quite such a fairy tale, although it could be described as an adventure. Savannah emailed to ask, 'Y'all getting spiritual and shit?' Well, only the shit bit really.

I went to the library. Sri Aurobindo's collected works occupied several shelves – he was definitely not a man of few words. There was no book less than 3 inches thick. I guess that being tucked away in his bedroom for twenty-four years gave him plenty of time to think and write. I picked up a *List of Publications for Beginners* that ran to nearly twenty books and two CD-Roms. I decided to try the promisingly titled *How Do I Begin?* by a disciple called Pandit, and another called *How Do I Proceed?* by the same man. Both were out on loan, with a waiting list. Pandit's *Dictionary of Sri Aurobindo's Yoga* was not on the reading list but was on the shelf. Despite the promising title it was still a little difficult to break down:

> *Aim of the Integral Yoga*: It is not merely to rise out of the ordinary ignorant world-consciousness into the divine consciousness, but to bring the supramental power of that divine consciousness down into the ignorance of mind, life and body, to transform them, to manifest the Divine here and create a divine life in Matter.

I wasn't quite sure which word to look up next but settled on 'Supramental', which, I discovered, was 'the direct self-existent Truth-Consciousness and the direct self-effective Truth-Power'.

This wasn't going to work. I decided to ask the Aurovilians I met to help me understand the key principles of Aurobindo's thinking, but unfortunately they were all in the same boat as me.

'What is Supramental Consciousness?' I asked a long-term official 'Master List' Aurovilian.

'I don't know. I never understood Sri Aurobindo. Don't tell anyone.'

'What about his epic poem, "*Savitri*"?'

'I don't know, I don't understand this either, but then even the Mother said she didn't understand much of it – and she'd read it twice. You know, most Aurovilians don't have time to sit and study, we are too busy working hard trying to make this place happen.'

I asked Bhaskar, the manager at Afsanah's, if he could shed any light on the poem. He rocked back in his executive chair, his feet not quite touching the ground. Crossing his fingers and addressing his comments to the ceiling, he said, sympathetically: '"*Savitri*" very, very difficult poem. Sri Aurobindo was Bengalian, Calcutta-born. When he was childhood he spent time in England. He spoke sixteen languages but he wrote "*Savitri*" in Bengali and then translated into English but not so easy. In Bengali easy. Otherwise very hard.' He rocked his chair back to an upright position and fixed me with his gaze – as a teacher to a slightly backward student. He spoke slowly. 'It's the story of a wife, Savitri, and her husband – Satyavan. Her husband dies, he is murdered. She is fighting with God. She needs her husband – very, very honest lady – she never look at another man. Finally she gets him back. In between there is lots of dialogue.' He looked at me as if that would be enough for one day. By way of explaining his expertise he told me, 'I am historian. Not only that, I learn English very quick – here in Auroville. I no need teacher. I just start to speak. I have many courses by correspondence. Not only that, I am M. Phil. Not only that, I am twenty-eight years. I am bachelor.'

I went to Savitri Bhavan for a talk on *The Synthesis of Yoga*, one of Sri Aurobindo's works. Sraddhalu, a Sri Aurobindo Ashram resident, resplendent in buttermilk silk *kurta pyjamas* gave the lecture. He discussed the content of two sentences for as many hours and I was none the wiser.

Fiddling with my scooter lights in the car park afterwards, I asked a fellow-seeker if she was having as much trouble as me.

'Sri Aurobindo is very complicated,' she admitted. 'He is leading you through one argument after another. You think, "Oh, that's his conclusion", and then he knocks it down. His mind worked in a special way. You only ever reach the real conclusion right at the end.'

I remembered Henri had told me that 'you read some and then you experience it and then "ahh – I see" and then some more. It is revealed slowly, when you are ready.'

I met an American artist who echoed this theme. She was holed up in the Green Belt teaching painting to people who couldn't draw a straight line, and was feisty – 'Who said the ability to draw a straight line is art anyway?' She told me that you bring in Supramental Consciousness 'by being open and conscious and patient. This awareness is key. You can't walk around saying, "I'm really open now," and expect something to happen immediately.'

I went to the Matrimandir quite regularly; although the acoustics were as bad as Osho's Auditorium, sitting in the circular marble chamber, on the white carpet, in mandatory white towelling socks, held a fascination for me. Just watching the seemingly heaven-sourced beams of white light cast a frosted crown over the big-ass crystal's glassy surface took the heat off my *chitta vritti*. Outside the red earth baked in the unrelenting sun; inside the mandir was cooled by some highly efficient air-conditioning. Unfortunately, the air-conditioning was the only thing I managed to draw down; Supramental Consciousness remained stubbornly supramental. I decided to follow the American artist's instruction and adopt a relaxed attitude to the unfurling of his wisdom. Supramental Consciousness would come when it was ready, but it might not be in this lifetime.

I had much more success discovering the joys of human unity – and since this was the Mother's stated intention for Auroville I was content, though I did feel a bit like the child at school whose report card says 'unacademic, but willing to take part'. There were plenty of places to unify with Auroville's humanity – although it only had 1,700 residents, the population of a village, it had the facilities of a large town. The noticeboard at the Solar Kitchen, Aurovilians' favourite lunch spot, advertised an eclectic mix of free entertainment and activities: from *The Last Samurai* to documentaries on US foreign policy; from crystal healing with Vijay at the Fertile Windmill to storytelling in the Tibetan Pavilion; from a Bengali dance night to Terry Pratchett's *The Wyrd Sisters*. Nothing for it but to jump in.

I went to see 'The Boys' playing on the roof terrace at the Solar Café. The café served up a welcome breeze alongside galettes, lobster, Russian chicken, melt-in-the-mouth chocolate cake and ginger tea (Auroville is teetotal), as two young guys from Bangalore took us on an old world musical tour – from Spain to Persia and Arabia. The audience ranged from three to sixty and from ageing hippies with *tundus* to Italian teenagers with braces and tight jeans straining over awkward hips. Several lifetimes of self-development courses were paying dividends on the dance floor; a shiny, happy woman radiant in crocheted white beanie hat, gossamer silk top and matching trousers shook her fifty-something booty, whilst younger things with belly piercings, revealed by low-slung tiered petticoats, brought good vibrations to their already perfectly tuned *manipura* navel *chakras*.

Auroville was no exception to the 'men watching from the sidelines' rule (Osho's resort was the only place I'd ever seen men as keen to dance as women). A thin Italian with a corkscrew mullet, high-waisted jeans and undone white trainers sat alongside his mate – a German with improbable blond hair combed forward over immense cheekbones – but even these men couldn't keep their inner selves hidden. Calvin Klein underwear peeped over the blond's jeans and the Italian's tiny white vest struggled to maintain adequate coverage over his Green Belt muscles.

At the Kosmos Café Earth Day Celebration, we sat in a circle on floor cushions in the Bharat Nivas pavilion and discussed sustainability. The convenor of the group, an eagle-eyed, long-haired thin fellow, handed a rubber globe to the man on his right and explained that only its possessor had the right to talk, and could we begin by defining 'sustainability'?

'My name is Gabriel. I am from Germany and my three-year-old told me yesterday "sustainability is keeping something for tomorrow".'

'My name is Michael. I am from Auroville. Sustainability is to create love.'

'My name is Brian. Sustainability is to sell as many solar panels as I can.'

I went for the classic approach and talked about the need to live in balance for the benefit of all parties. Everyone looked a bit nonplussed, then Bruce put it better than I did and got strong nods of agreement.

Then we moved onto the particular issues facing Auroville. The rubbery globe bounced around the room.

'Ten years ago Auroville was just push bikes, now there is money and the motorbikes have come.'

'The problem is the ego. We need to become part of the bigger consciousness. This is our yoga – we must sit with our fear, meditate on it, and understand what stops the self from participating in the collective consciousness. Until we understand this we will not progress.'

The rubbery globe passed into the hands of a striking, well-built girl of twenty, who was dressed head to foot in black and sat at the back of the room in an outer circle of latecomers. She sang Bob Marley's 'Jamming' and looked expectantly at the circle. The circle shifted uneasily and the ball bounced back into the inner circle, into my lap. I decided to get back onto more solid ground:

'I am a guest here so I don't know Auroville's issues in depth but I would like to suggest that the guesthouses encourage their visitors to be mindful of the amount of water they use, and perhaps laundry need not be done daily – as it is at Afsanah's.' There were some polite nods.

The rubbery globe bounced on. 'We must move from "*the* environment" to "*our* environment". This is where I am trying to shift my consciousness.' Everyone clapped. Why didn't I think of that? Bollocks. Bloody bollocks.

Too late to say anything original now – the eagle-eyed convenor was looking at the clock. 'It's six-thirty-three,' he said meaningfully. 'It's getting dark, we're running late, it's time for the music and that's where *we* are.'

The audience gathered, a good-looking array of strong shoulders and centred *manipura chakras* inside cheesecloth tunics and cropped trousers in the case of the men, and skimpy dresses in the case of the women. We settled down with giant samosas and mint tea to listen to a drumming circle of Tamil teenage boys, an improvization combining didgeridoo, maracas and drums, and a woman's recitation of a poem about wildness. This talk of wildness persuaded several small people in gingham skirts to come up to the stage and express themselves wildly. Two blond American boys played guitar and sang about the mysteries of life unravelling and people rising. They finished with a high five, a whoop and a big embrace. Pretty Francesca from Berlin told us, 'I have the big luck to play with Helge on violin and Matthew on piano.' Everyone clapped. 'We will spend the next forty-five minutes flying through the emotions of jazz.' Which we did.

Afterwards children with lions painted on their faces and silver tinsel wigs danced with their fathers, as their skimpily dressed mothers self-expressed on the vast expanse of grey slate floor. Young women with big bellies, dreamy eyes and creamy white skin lay on the floor in groups of three or four, heads drawn together in consultation, perhaps concerning the blond American boys. Another blond man, this one in a poncho and sombrero, lit up a *beedi* in the middle of the dance floor. I thought he was being rather charismatic but he was asked to leave immediately.

I had the most fun at the St Patrick's Day pub quiz. Perhaps it was because a rare drink was involved. Perhaps it was because it felt like human unity in action. Perhaps it was because of Spike.

I'd arrived in a really good mood – feeling inspired by the power of the Auroville fairy tale. Kalyan, who lived in Kuilapalayam, on the south-eastern border of Auroville, drove me the 5 kilometres down to the 'pub' – the Eden Garden restaurant just outside the teetotal Auroville perimeter. As we bounced over the township's potholes in his brand-new Ambassador, he explained why he loved living in Auroville: 'Auroville good place. Chennai live before – much tension, more expensive, very hard. Auroville life good. School good. House good. House Auroville five hundred rupees a month. Chennai same house one thousand eight hundred rupees. Auroville school, New Creation, fifty rupees a month. Chennai, same school three thousand five hundred rupees per quarter. Children fourteen, eleven, nine, eight, five and one. No more children. Fifteen years children. Wife thirty-six. Me thirty-nine. Children very happy. Our future very bright.' It was like talking to a smug Londoner who had moved to the countryside, except that Kalyan was entirely likeable.

Davina welcomed allcomers onto the rooftop of the 'pub'. Seeing I was alone (how sad), she put me in a higgledy-piggledy team, a collection of waifs and strays with no other place to go. There was a well-preserved fifty-something couple from the Home Counties – he was square-shouldered and chisel-jawed, his silver-grey hair cut in a soft modern style, and she was beyond thin, chain-smoking in an elegant black cocktail dress gathered at the halter-neck in soft folds, her fine black hair gathered behind her tiny ears. She became less and less coherent as the evening went on, fuelled, as we all were, by dyed green Kingfishers in lieu of Guinness. Sinead, a flame-haired Irish woman, could also knock them back, and did. Spike was born in the south Bronx and had recently moved to Zimbabwe where he wrote and directed plays with township kids. He was a man who knew the power of his smoked-wood African–American voice and playful smile, and wasn't afraid to use them. Rick was slightly less attractive to women – he had wild hair, a moustache, bad teeth and a very bad habit of nicking other people's Kingfishers.

As I hadn't had a drink for ten days, my bottle of Kingfisher went straight to my *nadis* – seriously affecting my ability to answer questions correctly, if at all. I do remember surprising myself by knowing that Pittsburgh was the American state named after a British prime minister, and that the Henry James novel turned into a film by Jane Campion was *Portrait of a Lady*, but then I let the side down by saying that Ilie Nastase was the first unseeded player to win Wimbledon when it was Boris Becker, and I couldn't help turn 1999 into Roman numerals despite it being a bit of a nerdy hobby at school.

We progressed onto the 'Star Turn' round in which one or all members of each team had to perform. A French man from 'The Little Green Men' played the flute badly. 'Sinn Fein' let Pam, a large-bosomed theatreland 'darling' with bright blonde hair, belt out 'Let's Do the Time Warp Again', complete with all the choreography. Sean from 'Guinness' recited an Irish poem three times before he got it right. There was the obligatory 'Danny Boy' and our team, 'The Rose of Tralee', sang 'Molly Malone' – for this we linked arms and swayed in the manner of drunk people. With the exception of Spike, who drank nothing stronger than pineapple juice, we didn't need to pretend.

Our performance in this round made up for the five points deducted by Davina from our team because she thought Spike was being mouthy. Spike got a lot of stick from the rest of the team until he reminded us that 'we should look to the umpire's motivation – she had chosen to create an issue out of the expression of an opinion'. We considered this grave political truth over our Kingfishers and had to agree that he was right. In general though, the participants played the game with the characteristic Aurovilian virtue of tolerance – despite the arbitrary decision-making. The Aurovilians joked that it seemed to be a microcosm of Auroville governance – in which several subcommittees would be consulted and the judge's decision would be final, based almost entirely on his or her own prejudice.

The final round, on all things Irish, carried double points. Thank goodness for Sinead – she turned out to be less drunk than the other Irish people there and answered every single question correctly, carrying us to an easy ten-point victory. We painted our faces green and red and held our prizes, pottery tankards made by Auroville craftspeople, proudly aloft. The losers, 'Sinn Fein', got potatoes. Spike whisked me around the makeshift dance floor, between the plastic chairs and bemused waiters, to Van Morrison's 'Bright Side of the Road'. I tried not to lose my flip-flops, or take the lead, but failed on both counts. I think Spike was looking for someone a little more polished, or at least less pissed. No matter. Sinead and I shared a taxi back to our guesthouses and entertained the driver with a reprise of 'Molly Malone'.

Sadly Spike hadn't given me his calling card but I met up with Sinead again the next day. She'd been invited to a birthday party in the fields of the Buddha Garden, a working farm offering accommodation in return for labouring in the fruit orchard, cashew plantation or chicken project. Volunteers worked from six till ten in the morning to qualify for an 80-rupee-a-night capsule looking out over the fields, or a 50-rupee bed in a mixed dorm. One of the capsules had burnt down the week before – they may have had a roof that 'lets through the cosmic vibrations and harmonizes your dreams' (according to an article in *Auroville Today* quoting the Aurovilian legend, Johnny – designer of the first capsule), but they weren't immune to careless incidents involving smoking.

We sat on big blankets amongst the long grass and wished upon shooting stars as we listened to Chris from Cambridge playing his guitar with a faraway look in his eyes. As the stars got brighter everyone lay top to toe – shaven heads, dreadlocks, bobs, plaits, pigtails, sensible heads. Fifty-five-year-olds, twenty-year-olds and one birthday girl – thirty-three years old today. Here we all were – human unity in action. Four Japanese women – Akiko, Hoshi, Midori and Suzu – cooked dinner for fifteen people, we ate noodles with sesame sauce, chocolate birthday cake and Aurovilian lemon star biscuits as Marcus from Germany gave a perfect recitation of 'Jabberwocky', and Lara, a Scottish friend of Akiko's, told me about gardening as meditation, living life according to yogic principles and her boyfriend's rubber fetish.

I was invited back to the Buddha Garden again a couple of days later for some early-morning Japanese yoga. Akiko, with her fringe, strong bone structure and headscarf, looked like a fifties land girl amongst the tall grasses. Over the next half an hour we tried to grow limber limbs and toned muscles instead of rocket leaves.

'In Japanese yoga we do thirty-two exercises to wake up all joints and muscles,' she explained. 'Begin like this.' She wiped the back of her palms across her cheeks, working her fingers underneath her eye sockets, palming her eyes and dropping her fists onto her forehead from a great height. 'Beautiful,' she said as she watched us pummel our foreheads. 'Feed your skull with your fingers.' She made fists and massaged into her groins, then down her legs and worked her way between the feet bones. 'What you call these?' she asked, pointing at the end of her feet.

'Toes,' said Lara helpfully.

'OK, pop toze.' She watched us do it. 'Beautiful.'

We slapped our legs and our chests with cupped palms and lay on our backs with the soles of our feet underneath our buttocks and tilted our knees up and down. That was surprisingly hard to do and actually hurt quite a lot on the baked earth. Japanese yoga may have been better named 'Slap and Tickle Yoga' owing to the curious mix of pleasure and pain, but the breakfast picnic that followed was all pleasure – locally baked bread, mango jam, honey, peanut butter and a homegrown rocket and tomato salad harvested the day before by Akiko herself. Her three friends joined us; we nodded, smiled and mispronounced each other's names – meet 'Luchi' and 'La'wa'.

I wondered what sequence of *asana* postures Sri Aurobindo and the Mother had cooked up for us in order to help us draw down Supramental Consciousness, but close scanning of the Solar Café noticeboard revealed no Auroville-branded yoga. I decided to try the classes at Pitanga, a body awareness centre in the eastern Residential

Zone, set up in 1991 by a Dutch yoga teacher and two Brazilian dancers. It was named after a sweet-smelling flowering bush native to South America that was symbolic of peace and harmony. Welcomed by a giant golden OM painted on the outside wall, I walked into an airy reception, complete with pond, ferns, atrium and a picture of the Mother. The yoga studio was a lovely light room with a polished cherry wood floor, but ropes hung along one wall and the shelves held neat rows of bolsters, blocks, blankets, straps and back racks. Pictures of Iyengar in scary positions lined the walls. Was I going to get shouted at again? Told to stretch my upper eyelashes?

I needn't have concerned myself. Sophie, a diminutive French woman with tight black curls, may have been Iyengar-trained but she was not in the militaristic school. We were gently guided through a slow afternoon class, the sun beating down as the fans whirred above us: 'Raise zee butox'; 'Make sure zee 'eels and toze are equally on zee floor'; 'Rotate zee pelvis'. We did some partner work in preparation for shoulder stand. Most of the other students were Aurovilian women with long, hard muscles who looked as if they could strangle a snake, but I was lucky and partnered one of the guys from the Buddha Garden party – a twenty-five-year-old shaven-headed, tattooed public school boy with whom I had lain on the blanket under the stars. We had to stand opposite each other, bend over at right angles as if we were bowing and touch our heads together, pressing our hands into each other's hot and sweaty backs to stretch out our spines. I can't imagine that this was supposed to be as sexy as it felt. Then we returned to an upright position, still facing each other, holding hands with arms outstretched and bending our knees, relying on each other for support as we went. He said I was helping him work on his trust issues. Anytime.

When I went back the next day, for another class, he was doing bare-chested t'ai chi in the wood outside the window. I found it very hard to concentrate.

I asked Kirsten, a European Aurovilian working at Pitanga, if there was any such thing as 'Auroville Yoga'. I'd read that the Mother had been very supportive of exercise – saying 'physical culture is the process of infusing consciousness into the cells of the body' – but Sri Aurobindo had been very specific in his view of *Hatha* yoga, and very much in agreement with Ramana Maharshi. It said in Pandit's *Dictionary of Sri Aurobindo's Yoga*:

> The chief processes of *Hatha* Yoga are *asana* and *pranayama* …
> The physical results – increased vitality, prolonged youth, health, longevity – are of small avail if they must be held by us as misers of ourselves apart from the common life for their own sake, not utilized, not thrown into the common sum of the world's activity. *Hatha* yoga attains large results, but at an exorbitant price and to very little purpose.

As Kirsten put it, rather more succinctly, 'If you do *Hatha* yoga for five hours a day what good are you in the world?' I wondered what Sri Aurobindo would have made of the *Ashtanga* students of Mysore and their dedication to winning the poolside best body contests.

The real yoga of Auroville, Kirsten explained, is the yoga of work, which 'is our tool; work is service – none of us came here to make money'. The emphasis was not what you did but the spirit in which you did it. 'There are no prestige jobs in Auroville,' she explained. 'When I first came I worked in the kitchens. I resisted it initially; I told myself that I didn't come here to work in a kitchen preparing food. And then I realized, and it took me nine or ten months to do so, that I was serving the community – after all, everyone needs to eat – and then I felt good about what I was doing.'

I asked her how people went about getting work here. Underneath the Solar Café's noticeboard was a Sri Aurobindo quote – 'Work done in true spirit is meditation'. There were opportunities to 'meditate' in the botanical gardens, in the kitchens, as a build supervisor, a project writer. Kirsten told me that 'in Auroville you must make your own work by asking around, making investigations. Newcomers will often try lots of new things and although they arrive thinking they will carry on with their old job in Auroville they often end up in something new ... there are fewer barriers. You can become a teacher here without the qualifications you would need in the West. There are a lot of new starts here ... Auroville gives you the space to feel who you are, to reflect on life and the self, to explore.' She admitted that all of this change and the lack of support and infrastructure inevitably meant that 'we get face to face with our shadow sides – individually and collectively ... there is a struggle before the transformation. We do what we do for the love of Auroville, not because it's easy. Actually it's very hard.'

I wasn't to be deterred. I was falling for this place, for this fairy tale land of sunshine, red lanes, big-ass crystals, tropical gardens and Gorgonzola cheese. I was considering staying for a while, becoming an official Newcomer, spending two years on probation, perhaps moving into the Salvador Dali house, definitely lying in my hammock, eating cheese and watching the fireflies. 'Have you got a job for me here?' I asked, only half-joking.

'Actually, Lucy, we do have an opening here at Pitanga,' said Kirsten. 'We have an exhibition here every two weeks and there is a lot of work with all the framing, hanging and displaying.'

'So,' I said slipping up a gear, into professional Londoner 'can do' mode, 'you need someone to sort it out, get the job done. No messing about.'

'Oh no,' said Kirsten, looking horrified, 'we need someone to work with the right attitude – with love and consciousness.'

No one had ever asked me to work with love and consciousness before, certainly not in my marge years, but maybe it was time to start.

~ 15 ~

'Atcha! OM! Boom!'

I decided to cancel the trip to Goa. I thought it would be a good idea to spend another week or two in human unity before making the full two-year Newcomer commitment. I wanted to talk to more long-term residents, delve deeper, and find out what life was really like on the Master List.

Unfortunately, the Master List weren't very interested in making friends with guests. I couldn't really blame them. Visitors were a daily disruption to the peace – arriving every day in huge coaches that made the otherwise quiet roads dangerous. In the short time I had been here I had learnt to avoid the main routes in and out of Auroville during Matrimandir visiting times. Bella, an Italian who had lived here for twenty years, told me with a resigned sigh, 'We surrender to the tourists.' Perhaps it was our transitory nature that put them off; I am not sure I would have bothered with people who were only staying for a week or two, and what chance did I have when even those Newcomers who had made the two-year commitment were having trouble gaining acceptance?

I stayed behind after one of the Savitri Bhavan talks to chat to a middle-aged lady with a worried expression and a bob. She told me how hard it had been to settle in Auroville when she first arrived six years ago: 'The Aurovilians were not very friendly. There was so much aggression – it was "give me this", "give me that" – no helping at all. You just had to go and get on with it. Today it is better but it is still a struggle.' She still seemed to be upset by the experience and I wasn't sure it really had got a lot better.

Glen, an official Newcomer, told me about the difficulties he'd been having: 'I am not allowed to leave for two years. If I do go I must tell the Newcomer board, and now I have been a Newcomer for longer than that because I have been out of Auroville a lot. The Master List tell me, "It's no good – you are not an Aurovilian", but *they* are going out of Auroville all the time – many are out for the whole summer, for four months at a time.'

Perhaps the Newcomers were being punished for having things too easy – after all, the original pioneers had created enchanted woods out of barren deserts with their bare hands – but if this was true, it seemed a little unfair. The Newcomers couldn't help their timing, they seemed to be committed to trying to live a different way – and importantly, every Newcomer I met put his money where his mouth was. Glen gave back to Auroville two-thirds of the money he earned – a high rate of tax on a low income. He told me that nobody gets very well paid in Auroville so lots of people supplement their income by earning money outside, and many still had homes elsewhere. It didn't surprise me that two-thirds of Newcomers left within three years; what was more surprising was Glen's continuing dedication. 'Are you sure it's worth it?' I asked him.

'When I am here I get pissed off, then I go somewhere else and know Auroville is where I want to be. I have been to many places in the world and this is the one that gives me the space, the nature that I love.'

The space he was speaking of had nothing to do with where he and his family lived. This was another area of apparent inequality. Glen said he couldn't imagine that he would ever have the same housing privileges as Master List Aurovilians – as more people entered the township the pressure on housing grew. No Salvador Dali house for him; instead his family were housed in a tiny flat in a soulless apartment block.

Glen wasn't the only Newcomer having trouble with property. I came across Fritz the Farmer on my travels through the Green Belt. He was sitting on his veranda drinking some extra strong coffee, and asked me to join him for a cup. It emerged that he was involved in a boundary dispute with his neighbour. Both parties had agreed to erect a fence, they just couldn't agree on the size or materials. Fritz favoured a cheaper, simpler option and had moved forward on this. He told me, 'I am the faster worker so I will put up my fence first.' He showed me the wooden fence and added, thoughtfully, 'I know that his workers will steal my produce so I have instructed my workers to steal his first.' Perhaps this wasn't quite the fairy tale I had imagined.

Later on that same afternoon I picked up a copy of the township's official newspaper, *Auroville Today*. I was about to discover that, like all fairy tales, Auroville had a shadowy underbelly; that conflict and even occasionally extreme violence, were actually as much a part of the Auroville story as the enchanted wood.

The March issue of the paper was dedicated to the memory of Sydo, a 41-year-old Dutch Aurovilian murdered in his house. He had joined Auroville in 1996 to live and work in the Green Belt and his picture showed him to be typical of the laid-back guys that I had admired hard at work in the forest. He sounded great fun – a free-spirited clown playing the flute in the enchanted wood, loved by children for his jokes and good nature. *Auroville Today* speculated that he was killed because he was the key witness in a robbery at his neighbour Steve's house, which had left him and Steve in hospital, slashed by knives and *katthies* (bill-hooks.) Sydo had positively identified a gang of Tamil villagers as responsible for the robbery, and the available evidence suggested that they might have returned to his house in Udumbu to brutally murder him in the dead of night.

The relationship between Auroville and the Tamil villages bordering the township's land was a difficult one. The problems had begun, as Henri described, when the Sri Auribindo Society had hired *goondas* to scare Aurovilians off the land. Life in these 'backward and in need of development' villages was already turbulent, without throwing a major East/West culture clash into the mix. The *Auroville Today* reports of village tensions – gang-related killings, assaults and robberies whipped up by feuds between modern political governance and the old-fashioned ways of the temple and the elders – read like plot lines for *The Godfather*. In Tamil culture, family honour is everything. Throw into this smouldering cauldron the exposure of the primarily *gounder* caste (labourers) and *harijans* to Aurovilian Westerners riding big motorbikes, living in even bigger houses and, in the case of the women anyway, wearing skimpy *manipura-chakra*-revealing dresses – somewhat at odds with the 6 metres of fabric worn by Tamil lady folk – and it's not surprising that human unity would find difficulty expressing itself. I found it hard to imagine the peaceful people I met around Auroville going home to participate in the unfolding of these *Godfather* plots in their villages. They always seemed so friendly and gentle – more so than the Westerners, actually. Male friends strolled, warm hand in warm hand, and helped me fix the lights on my scooter; the women managed to grin at me even as I hurtled towards them on 50ccs of uncontained power.

Whatever the truth of the relationship between Westerners and Tamils, human unity was not evident in the distribution of housework around the township – I didn't see any white faces watering gardens or doing the laundry. The Buddha Garden gang were unimpressed.

'It's colonial,' said Lara.

'It's disgusting,' said Akiko.

Akiko was doing her bit – making hammocks alongside Tamil teenage girls – but she was struggling with cultural differences in the pace of work. 'The Japanese are taught to work hard – to focus on the job,' she said. 'The Tamil people are very slow – they have not been taught in our way.'

I wondered whether, with such differences, this utopian experiment was ever going to work, but arguably, desperate for foreign investment, India needed it to work more than anywhere else in the world.

I was, of course, also on the lookout for some 'one-to-one' human unity; I had high hopes of finding my prince in the enchanted wood. There seemed, on paper at least, plenty of potential soulmates. There were 710 men here out of 1,304 adults, and they seemed the right sort.

Bella told me, over a cappuccino in the Solar Café, that 'the community is very creative – we are artists, musicians, writers and we are creating solar panels also'. So plenty of action, right? Bella looked sad and somewhat resigned to her single status. 'We are like everyone else. It is lonely sometimes – it can be hard. I would have preferred to be more social but it's not happening and meanwhile I have plenty of self-work to do.'

I found the idea of self-work of any kind rather depressing – I felt there had been too much of that kind of thing back in my London flat.

Fritz explained, as he drove the stakes of his fence into the ground, that 'no one in Auroville stays with the same person for long'. He explained that there wasn't much emphasis on making relationships work and that 'the Mother didn't think people should have to stay together if they weren't in love. She didn't really support marriage – she said, "if you are not beyond marriage then marry" but she thought it was all a bit childish. Actually though,' Fritz grinned, 'she was married to a diplomat and had two children, her grandson is somewhere here in Auroville.'

It began to dawn on me that Auroville was a place for people who valued independence more than relationships. The feisty 'I can do it on my own' spirit was evident everywhere – from the photos Henri showed me, to the single girls on big motorbikes, to the kind of courses on offer. There were plenty of therapies for individuals – crystal healing, polarity work and pranic healing – but very little in the way of group work. Perhaps, as it was such a small community, it would have been dangerous to unload too much personal stuff; Osho-style cathartic convulsions in the centre of the therapy room, as people confessed to terrible childhood tragedies and re-birthed, probably wouldn't sit well alongside the need to get on with harvesting the cashew nuts the next day.

Feeling disappointed, I decided to pay the Buddha Garden another visit. I'd found lots of evidence of human unity under its stars last week, but it seemed things had changed since then and even Akiko, with her US Masters in Peace Studies, was having a hard time. Two of the ten Buddha Garden volunteers were turning in just one hour of work a day, not doing any of the cooking and eating everyone else's food. It seemed straightforward enough to me. 'Why don't you just tell them to get off their butts?' I asked her.

'Ahh, because we have no rules here. I have to wait until they have awareness of their actions, and how long is that going to take?'

'I think you might be waiting a while,' I guessed.

'Yes, so now I just take my food and eat alone in my capsule. I am not cooking for anyone else.'

I had been thinking about moving into the Buddha Garden, becoming Akiko's next-door neighbour (once they'd rebuilt the burnt-out capsule) but it was beginning to sound like the isolationist life I'd led in London. All I needed was a Café Culture ready meal and a colour telly and I would be back where I started.

My increasing sense of disenchantment was making me feel distinctly off-balance when, in the course of one day, I broke my sunglasses, dropped my camera, spilt water over my mobile and left my watch on the beach.

I went to see Sophie for some retuning. I'd been imagining another delicious round of long slow partner work, perhaps with that tattooed English guy – but she was on tough form, and he wasn't there. We did four types of balancing our arms on our knees, the emphasis on the mechanics of the pose: 'Level zee buttox, Lucie, feel zee bodee.' We did three types of balancing on one leg: '*Plus fort*, Sylvie. *Les jambs*, Josef.' Then we hung upside down on ropes: '*Oui*, Sylvie. *Très bien*, Sylvie.' There was no '*très bien*, Lucie', and I found myself longing once again for a flow-based class in which I could lose myself.

I met Glen for a late breakfast. I told him, over eggs and roast bread (the toaster at Afsanah's had broken yet again), about my bad technology day and my disappointment in discovering that the fairy tale might have a dark side. He smiled sympathetically. 'On days like this you must just laugh, surrender to the will of the universe.'

'What do you think is wrong?'

He paused for a moment and looked thoughtful. 'One of your three bodies must be out of alignment.'

'My three bodies?'

'Yes, each body has a vibration which corresponds with different levels of consciousness. There is the body you know – your *sthula sharira* or physical body – waking consciousness, which is discarded when you die. But beneath that is your *sukshma sharira*, your astral body – it can fly in space through the astral universe and it's where your *chakras* are located. Channelling and clairvoyance occur through this body, *devas* – heavenly beings – tend to get stuck here, they get intoxicated by the giddy pleasures of the astral realms, but these pleasures are illusory and the real bliss is to be found in the third body – the *karana sharira*. This is the location of the soul, the higher Self, pure consciousness. I don't know which of your bodies is out of alignment but I suggest that you create a pranic egg to protect yourself.'

I ate my omelette thoughtfully. 'How do I do that?'

'Just lie down and imagine yourself surrounded by *prana*; it is enveloping you, like an egg.'

I was a bit unsure about the precise methodology involved in creating such an egg but fortunately Lara popped round for a chat. She'd also studied pranic eggs and offered to help out. I lay on the grass next to my hammock and closed my eyes. She spoke slowly.

'In creating a pranic egg you are protecting yourself for the day, creating an envelope around yourself – spinning three layers of protection. First meditate on your aura – did you know it's four inches thick?' I didn't. 'Breathe. What colour is your aura, Lucy? Orange? Purple? Red?' I decided it was white and shimmering, like gossamer angel wings. 'Now think about your physical body. Feel the connection between the body and the air. Breathe.' We moved on to the *sukshma sharira*, the astral body. 'Visualize each one of the *chakras* as you move up the body – from the root, the *muladara*, to *sahasra padma*, your cosmic *chakra*. Breathe. What colour is each *chakra*? Meditate on each one, protect it, breathe into it.

'Now let's move towards the core of your being, towards *karana sharira*. Know that you are *sat-chit-ananda*. Existence-consciousness-bliss. Can you feel the bliss warming your skin?' My skin did indeed feel hot – more likely the action of the sun than bliss absolute, however.

Lara left me to breathe for a few minutes whilst she went to the loo. When she came back she was businesslike. 'And there you are,' she said, as if she was serving up a Starbucks coffee, 'ready for the day.'

I thanked her. I felt calmer but the real beneficiary was my mobile – it was working for the first time since I'd doused it with water. Perhaps my three bodies had also been retuned. Lara suggested that I go to the Fertile Windmill to get some crystals to guard against further upset.

The blackboard outside the windmill's so-called 'OM Hut' read:

Sirius Crystal Shrine.
Encounter yourself at your own door.

Here we can
If you're so inclined
Find your personal stone
Reveal everything about yourself that you never wished to know.
Meditate and become
Enlightened together
Go always beyond.

As there was no one manning the shrine I enquired about booking an encounter with myself in the shop, but I was told that the shrine's CEO was away for two weeks. I could choose my own crystal with the help of a 200-page guide but it seemed to boil down to choosing the one that spoke to you. Fearing a repeat of the Rishikesh sapphire and diamonds affair, I decided to risk relying on my pranic egg – it seemed to be working.

Bad decision. An hour later I ran out of scooter juice. By the time I'd hitched a ride to the gas station on the other side of the township and hitched another ride back, I was very glad that I had a session booked with Henri. When I arrived, the living fairy tale was talking in fluent Tamil to a villager with a bad shoulder. I gave the villager some Aurovilian cookies in the hope that they would speed his recovery, and retired to the 'temple'.

Henri watched me perform my Somatics exercises, which I had been doing every day and which did seem to be making a difference. He was pleased. 'Atcha. The body is responding. The consciousness is returning – it is speaking to you. Listen to what it is saying. Nothing to fear.' He began the massage; my body's responses were met with the usual appreciation: 'Atcha! OM! Boom!'

I asked him to tell me the story of how he had come to live in the enchanted wood. 'I lived in the ashram until nineteen seventy-seven,' he said. 'I'd been doing a lot of work with the Aurovilians and they kept asking me, "When are you going to come?" One day I went to work at Auroville as usual and once again someone asked me, "When are you coming?" I replied, "I don't know, maybe tomorrow, maybe in a year." But there we were having lunch, that same day, and something happened. In that moment I knew – *now* I must come. So I went back to the ashram to tell them. I left ten days later – I had to leave a bit of time so as not to make too much mess for them. And then I arrived and I didn't know where I was going to stay, then someone said to me, "Someone has just left Aspiration," and so I went immediately. I got on my bicycle with my things – and boom! There I was. That was it – in that moment. That is how it must be – the mind working, always thinking, this way, that way and then … Boom! We must live in the moment always.'

Glen had told me that Henri had met the Dalai Lama. I wanted to know what happened when two enlightened beings shook hands.

'I had seen him once before at a distance,' said Henri. 'He had come to visit the Mother at the ashram. I saw him with crowds of other people. Then, many years later, I was in Auroville giving a massage and my friend said, "Do you want to come and be part of the group that meets the Dalai Lama?" And my mind did not waver. "Yes!" I said. Boom! And then we met and we hugged and he said, "You are just like me," and we smiled and laughed and we walked arm in arm to the Matrimandir. As we hugged, I could feel something very special – something peaceful and quiet. The mantra *"OM Mani Padme Hum"* came to me – it used to be in my mind a lot. I told this to him and he smiled. OM.'

I decided to tell this enlightened being about my frustrated attempts to merge with cosmic bliss, to discover my Eternal Self, my search for *sat-chit-ananda*. 'I am confused,' I said. 'Every time I think I have found it, it disappears. I thought this place was a fairy tale, and now I have discovered that it's not. You know, I don't think I know what I am searching for any more.'

'Ah,' he smiled, 'the search for the Divine. But there is no need to search. It is inside of you. Did you know that your body is the Divine in matter?'

I explained that I'd been told that this was so but I was looking for hard evidence.

He replied, 'You cannot describe it – it is not a thought process – it is something you can only experience. It is the thing that is bigger than all of us. The thing that is in all of us – you, me, him, her, the trees. In each moment we are in union with the universal. Just be – that is all. It is so vast.' He expanded his arms as if to embrace the whole world. 'Knowing this thing exists makes the world expand – we are not separated from each other. I am the same as you. In this there is peace. Stop reaching for the goal, live in this moment. In this there is power. You will know what to do.'

As I walked to my scooter I wiped the tears from my eyes. Once again I had that feeling of leaving the flotsam and jetsam of my hopes and fears behind, of sinking to the ocean bed – the experience that I'd had at Ramanasramam – of finding a stillness, an awareness of a bigger reality, a place without ego, hatred, cravings, uncertainty and misapprehension, that was both within me and outside of me.

Ten minutes later I was hurling a pile of clean laundry at the wall. The merger with cosmic bliss hadn't lasted long. When I got back to Afsanah's I'd found lots of lovely freshly ironed clothes on the chair outside my room, but my beloved Paul and Joe jeans were missing in action, presumed dead. Bollocks. Bloody bollocks. I'd found myself insisting that the unfortunate Bhaskar go through the entire guest laundry cupboard to find them, and shouting, 'What am I supposed to wear now?' when they didn't turn up.

Those pesky *kleshas* were certainly giving my flawless diamond of a mind another pounding. There I was, in a state of total *asmita*, falsely identifying myself with a bit of denim. I had to laugh. But actually it was no laughing matter; it wasn't funny at all. Of course the jeans weren't important, and I apologized immediately to Bhaskar. But my over-reaction did make me wonder what I'd been doing these last five months. Forcing myself to calm down and think about it, I realized that I had made little progress since the day I had stood at the taxi rank in Delhi and shouted at the drivers and porters. Despite a few brushes with cosmic bliss – in Vinay P. Menon's yoga class, in an enchanted wood and in the *darshan* hall of a man who had been dead for more than fifty years – I hadn't moved with any degree of permanence beyond materialism and make-up. What's more, I was bored of ricocheting from one extreme emotion to another, with living out of a suitcase. I missed my family and I missed the Cappuccino Gurus. I was really exhausted, with travelling from one end of the country to the other, with the effort of having to keep going, with trying to be a good student, with making new friends, with trying to find my guru and life's deeper meaning, with squeezing what should have been several lifetimes' work into a few months.

I lay in my hammock and stared fiercely at the fireflies and the fairy lights glowing softly in the rhododendron bushes. Why hadn't I made any progress? Was Beckle right? He'd noticed the 'OM Yoga' T-shirt I'd been wearing in class – brought back for me by a friend from Cyndi Lee's yoga studio in New York – and we'd got into a conversation about the large number of yoga schools I had visited. 'When I saw that T-shirt I thought to myself, "That girl's just shopping",' he'd said jokingly. Except that it wasn't a joke at all.

Had the whole five months just been one long shopping trip – collecting experiences without changing on the inside, where it counted? There was plenty of evidence for Beckle's case. The shopping list had consisted of a new life, a better body, some deeper meaning and a boyfriend, and a list of places, yoga schools, where I might find them. When I thought about it, there wasn't much difference between this and an afternoon's shopping back home. If I didn't find what I wanted in Joseph, I'd move on to Selfridges and Whistles. My immediate instinct, when I'd identified with Frenchy's beauty school predicament in *Grease*, was to leave KYM – to find new 'shops'. But I couldn't go on shopping indefinitely, and what were my motivations anyway? Where was all of this leading? Wasn't it all an escape from real life? An indulgence? And, assuming that I ever succeeded, what would be the practical benefit of being an 18 per cent body fat Yoga Goddess, sipping mango juice in an ashram hammock 4,000 miles from home? Wasn't this an escapist fantasy? If none of the schools on the list delivered the goods, then what? Would I disappear off up the mountain, sit with ash-smeared *sadhus*, their matted hair wild and abandoned, as I performed austerities – holding my arm above my head for twelve years until it shrivelled and my nails grew 3 feet? Somehow, I couldn't see it. It was time to stop shopping. It was time to call it a day. The quest was over.

The turnaround I was looking for wasn't going to be wrought by enrolling at another yoga school, the acquisition of more OM T-shirts, yoga books or laminated yellow certificates. I needed to change my perspective. I remembered something one of the Cappuccino Gurus had said. We'd met in Café Seventy-Nine, and she'd come straight from a course where she was studying the so-called 'Paradoxical Theory of Change'. She told me that change occurs only when we become what we truly are, not when we are trying to be something we are not. Change can't happen when we are trying to escape our true nature. If I'd learnt anything I had learnt that; unfortunately, when you travel you take yourself with you. Perhaps if I could just accept myself as I was and stop trying to be extraordinary, stop trying to be a Yoga Goddess, I would actually make some progress. It also struck me that the most inspirational people I had met in India – MP, Mr Hospitality, Henri, the students Menaka introduced us to at KYM – were so-called 'ordinary' people, waiters, railway workers, government employees, tailors, masseurs, teachers. In fact, Georg Feuerstein remarked that it seemed to him that the closer people got to Self-Realization the more ordinary they became.

When I thought about these 'ordinary' people, the reason I found them so inspiring was because their yoga practice stretched way beyond their mat. They saw yoga as a state of mind, an attitude to life, and the world as their school. Yoga was, for all of them, 'a harmonious way of living', not a one-off physical goal – they knew that all they had to do was look within. Enlightenment was not a trophy to be lifted high in one triumphant moment, it was about trying to increase the moments of seeing clearly, and choosing wisely in daily life. None of them seemed to want a yoga calendar body. None of them seemed interested in balancing on a rock in handstand. For them yoga was not a huge topic of conversation, unless a Westerner asked about it. It was an unremarkable thing – *pranayama*, meditation and perhaps a few simple sun salutations. It was practised informally, not in a big class on the instructions of a big name teacher, but at home – quietly, without fuss. MP had conducted his daily devotional *puja* to Ganesh at home before his thirteen-hour day at the Madras Café began. Handsome Kedarnarth, the man on the train to Chennai, had taken his 'upside downing' like a gin and tonic at the end of the day. He didn't see any need to deprive himself of the real thing shortly thereafter. Neither did he see any need to wear orange, white or even maroon (unless he had a particular urge), and he certainly saw no need to leap up and down a blue sticky mat for three hours a day.

The thing that really distinguished these 'ordinary' people was their ability to celebrate the ordinary, to take pleasure in everyday life, to wonder at small things. Their happiness, their *santosha* or contentment wasn't spoilt by excessive *raga*, or desire for material wealth. Their day didn't start with 'If only …' They didn't feel that they needed a trip to Joseph, or an OM T-shirt in order to be happy. Their happiness was right here, right now, in this place, wherever 'this place' happened to be. MP was happy as long as he was doing his best for his family, his customers and his fish. Mr Hospitality's only desire was to serve God, showing visitors his favourite ashram and its beautiful surroundings. Mohan, Taresh and Akshay were happy doing anything, as long as it involved an Elvis soundtrack, a rickshaw and some pink tinsel.

If being this 'ordinary' could make you this happy, this content, I wanted in. It was time to ditch the big goals – they weren't really getting me anywhere (interesting that if we reverse the 'o' and the 'a' in 'goal', we get 'gaol') and start with some small stuff. I would give up on trying to make headlines – the big merger with cosmic bliss, the quest for bodily perfection, the recruiting of a retinue of male followers – and I would definitely stop trying to stand on my head, which hurt too much. Instead I would concentrate on the small print – trying to increase the moments of seeing clearly and choosing wisely in everyday life, just like my 'ordinary' gurus.

My life in India had been a mass of contradictions; one minute I was beyond materialism and sleeping on an inch-thick mattress, the next I was dropping £130 in Amethyst. One minute I was sipping coconut juice between classes and discussing the yoga *sutras*, the next I was swigging Pinot Grigio with Liv, Johan, Beckle, Harley, Savannah and Roxanne on the Park Hotel's roof terrace. One minute I was considering life as a Swoony Swami orange-robed sunbeam, the next I was sunning myself in a bikini on a Keralan beach. India had exposed these contradictions before my eyes, and I knew that yoga wouldn't help me erase them, nor would it stamp out life's challenges, kill all known *kleshas* dead (actually I didn't really want to stamp out life's challenges anyway – who wants to operate their toy ship from the shores of a boating lake when they can ride the ocean's waves?), but it could help me make better decisions, establish more equilibrium, slow down a bit. I was learning in my *asana* practice not to get bound up in what I could or couldn't do, but just 'to be', to be aware, to be content with where I was. I would try to live my life the same way.

There was a lot I would miss about India. I had fallen in love with the place and its people – the gentle folk of Rishikesh – so full of grace, the Himalaya, the Ganges, the endless blue skies, the orange robes, the incense, the *kumkum* and the *pujas*, but I was ready to go home. I would redirect my energies, change the way I lived. I didn't want to become an 'Eco Yogi' – living in a log cabin in the Cornish woods, without mains electricity or a washing machine, hanging out on my veranda like the good ladies of the Auroville Green Belt, with their unshaven legs and untamed bosoms. My self-acceptance programme would begin with the first step – admitting that I was a 'Cappuccino Yogi' and that my spiritual homeland was north London. I would reinstate myself in Café Seventy-Nine and Café Violette, and try to put yoga's ancient teachings into practice, both on and off the mat.

How would I make a living? The world of advertising was certainly looking a lot less crazy than some of the worlds I'd just inhabited. After all, there was nothing much more ordinary than a tub of margarine. And I had to admit that I felt more at home in the presence of singing sunflowers and advertising folk than Gucci gurus and Hugging Mothers. Understanding why sunflowers made people feel happy, especially when they sang, had regained its fascination. And I'd always got a lot of satisfaction out of the work I did on government campaigns like tobacco education – it made me very happy to think that I might have played some small part in helping smokers to give up. I also wanted to write – Mrs P, the astrologer in Rishikesh, had been very firm in her prediction that I would write a book on yoga and foreign travel and I had really enjoyed keeping a record of my journey. *What* I did was beginning to seem less important than *how* I did it. I would definitely try to work with a sense of equanimity and contentment, and with the love and consciousness that Kirsten had made such an important condition of hanging pictures at Pitanga.

Living in this new way wouldn't be without its challenges; I suspected that there would be hourly falls from grace, but the benefit of my Indian shopping trip was that my bags were now bursting with yogic weaponry (I was, after all, supposed to be that fiery, full-of-rage goddess Durga, who annihilated entire armies with her ten arms). I had chanting – which I'd begun to enjoy so much it was regularly taking me to the state of *mudita*. I had been hugged by a Hugging Mother, I had my twelve 'OM *shanties*', I knew how 'to be' in an *asana*, I'd followed Savannah's example and come home with a suitcase full of Maroma's

'Yoga', 'Happy Heart', 'Joy' and 'Inner Peace' aromatherapy shower gels and shampoos, I had a picture of the Swoony Swami dancing on Christmas Eve, and I had my KYM orange *dhurrie*. I could meditate on my new 'ordinary' gurus – the KYM students, Henri, MP and Mr Hospitality – and I could freedive my way to the peace and tranquillity of the ocean bed. I could even fake a *Tantric* orgasm, though in general terms I didn't want to be faking anything from now on. Hopefully I wouldn't need to – I had that sapphire and diamonds ring which was going to bring my future husband to me, provided I meditated on it on Thursdays, or was it Tuesdays?

OK, so I wasn't going home a Yoga Goddess wearing a shiny 'new and improved' sticker. To all intents and purposes I'd failed on my quest – but I didn't feel like a failure. I actually felt happy and optimistic. Failure had set me free. I'd given up on perfection and I didn't feel beholden to the demands of my ego any more. If I lay very still in my hammock I thought I could detect once more the vague whisperings of that ancient Eternal Self – telling me that in breaking free of the self-imposed goal, or gaol, without the ego's fear of failure, I would find the world to be a bigger place.

So I crossed the remaining yoga schools off my list – I had what I needed now, no need for any more shopping – and headed back to London to meet up with the Cappuccino Gurus. I already knew what they would say – was I finally getting in touch with my own inner guru? The one that says be content with what you have. The one that says happiness is always available to us, we just have to look inside ourselves. The one that says there is perfection in imperfection. The one that says talk to men on trains. The one that says eat M&S chocolate peanuts and be blissful. The one that says possess only what is necessary – and necessary may include pretty dresses, though they don't always need to be labelled Joseph. The one that says life is a delicate balancing act: one-part mugs of Maharishi Ayur-Ved Calming *Vata* Tea and standing on one-leg yogic tree poses; one-part bottles of Pinot Grigio and falling over.

Recipe for Apple Muffins

With thanks to the Downs Syndrome Association of Tamil Nadu and my mum – who roadtested the recipe for me in an English country kitchen, and to Oliver (my stepfather) for selflessly trying the first batch. According to Mum's email:

> He did this without demur, was heroic in the face of such a taxing task, composed himself with due reverence and dropped quite a few crumbs on the floor in the cause of progress. He liked them and had two last night (secretly, he thinks).

Peel and core three medium cooking apples (enough to fill a 350ml cup twice) and chop them into a small saucepan. Add two tablespoons of caster sugar, quarter of a cup of water and half a teaspoon of cinnamon. Cook gently together till soft, smoothing out any lumps with a fork. Leave to cool in the pan.

Stir these dry ingredients together in a bowl:

One cup of oats
Quarter cup of raisins
One tablespoon of milk powder
One and a half cups of self-raising flour
Half a cup of caster sugar
One teaspoon of baking powder
Half a teaspoon of baking soda

Add 4 tablespoons corn oil to one cup of water and mix. Add to dry ingredients, mixing in. Add chopped and cooled apple mush and mix well again.

Fill paper cases three-quarters full with the mixture and put cases into a muffin tray. Cook for approximately 20–25 minutes at 170°C, (160°C for fan-assisted ovens) or Gas Mark 3.

Allow to cool for ten minutes. Lift out and place on wire rack to cool some more, if you can wait. Eat before anyone else does!

Glossary

Abhinivesa – excessive attachment to material and physical life

Adho mukha vrksasana – handstand

Advaita Vedanta – literally means 'not two', representing a monistic or non-dualistic Hindu system in which the individual Atman or Self is a part of Brahman

Ahimsa – non-violence, respect for all living things

Ajna chakra – the mind *chakra*, located at the third eye between the eyebrows

Amrita – the nectar of immortality

Anahata chakra – the air chakra, located at the heart centre

Ananda – bliss

Apanasana – knees are pulled into the chest on the exhale and moved away to full arms extension on the inhale

Aparigraha – detachment from possessions and desires

Arati Prayer – the 'Prayer of Light'

Asana – yoga postures that regulate the physical body, promoting concentration

Ashram – Hindu retreat for the pursuit of a spiritual life

Ashtanga yoga – the eight limbs of yoga, also the dynamic *Hatha* yoga system developed by Krishnamacharya and now taught by his student Sri K. Pattabhi Jois in which the practitioner moves through a sequence of poses on the breath. Movement through the sequence creates heat which burns toxins and creates a flexible, toned and healthy body

Asmita – false identification with the immediately experienced self, egoism

Avatar – the visible manifestation of a Hindu deity

Avidya – misapprehension, ignorance

Ayurveda – a *Vedic* system of balanced health for mind, body and spirit

Bandha – physical locks that help to direct *agni* or fire, to any waste matter that may block the flow of prana

Beedi – tobacco tightly wrapped in olive green leaves and tied with thread

Bhagavad Gita – 'the Lord's Song', one of the fundamental sources of Hindu philosophy in which Krishna explains to Arjuna the nature and purpose of human life and points Arjuna in the direction of *Jnana*, *Karma* and *Bhakti* yoga

Bhagwan – the blessed one, Lord (also spelt Bhagavan)

Bhajan – Hindu devotional song

Bhakti yoga – the yoga of love and devotion

Bikram yoga – a vigorous sequence of postures designed by Bikram Choudhury, practised in a room heated to 100°F/38°C to promote sweating, weight loss, the burning of toxins and flexibility

Brahma – one of the trinity of Hindu gods, Brahma is the creator of the universe

Brahmacharya – purity and sexual restraint

Brahman – universal cosmic consciousness, the ultimate whole

Brahmin – the highest caste of Hindu society, traditionally eligible for the priesthood

Buddha – literally 'the awakened one', the ninth *avatar* of Vishnu for Hindus

Bujangasana – 'cobra pose': stomach and palms on the ground, upper body raised, looking straight ahead

Chai – Indian tea made with milk, sugar and spices

Chakra – seven wheels of vital energy located in the astral body along the *sushumna*

Char Dam – the four 'starting points' that are regarded by Hindus as holy shrines: Badrinath; Kedarnarth; Gangotri; and Yamunotri

Chaturanga dandasana – 'four-limbed staff pose': a press-up position in which the body is held parallel to the floor

Chillum – a clay pipe with a narrow funnel, used to smoke weed

Chit – consciousness

Chitta – the mind

Chitta vritti nirodhah – the second yoga sutra, meaning controlling or stilling the activities of the mind, so that the true Self can be seen without distortion

Darshan – an audience with a spiritual master

Darshana – literally 'ways of seeing', the six principal strands of Hindu philosophy, of which yoga is one

Devi – the supreme Hindu mother goddess, worshipped in lots of forms including Shakti, Durga and Kali

Dharana – concentration of the mind, one-pointedness

Dhoti – a long cloth worn by Hindu men around the waist, usually white, which can be worn pulled up between the legs

Dhurrie – traditional heavy Indian rug

Dhyana – meditation

Dosha – Literally means 'fault'. In Ayurveda the diagnosis of disease is done by balancing the three different energies in the body – these energies are called *dosha*

Duhkha – distress, suffering, sadness, the result of ignorance

Durga – the unconquerable form of Devi, a beautiful but fierce, independent warrior Goddess, traditionally depicted with a golden body, riding a lion or tiger, slaying a buffalo demon, her ten arms holding her weapons, jewels and rosaries

Dvesa – aversion, repulsion, rejecting people or experiences because they have brought pain in the past

Dvipada pitham – 'half bridge pose': upper back on the floor, knees bent, buttocks raised

Eka pada rajakapotasana – 'one-legged king pigeon pose': sitting upright, one foot is folded into the groin, other leg out behind and bent at the knee, the foot of which is held towards the forehead as the back arches

Eternal Self – the Seer or *purusha*, a Self that is changeless and stable, separate from the Seen; or *prakriti*, the ever-changing mind, body and emotions, all matter

Ganesh – elephant-headed god, invoked to remove obstacles and bring good luck

Garudasana – 'eagle pose': balancing on one leg, wrapping the opposite leg around the back of the other ankle, mirroring this action with entwined arms, resting one elbow on top of the other and wrapping one arm around the back of the other whilst pressing the palms together

Giri pradakshina – a 14-kilometre pilgrimage circuit of Arunachala hill

Goonda – hired thug or bully

Guru – from *gu*, darkness and *ru*, illumination, therefore a guru is a master who illuminates his students' darkness

Halasana – 'plough pose': lying on the top of the shoulders, arms and feet over the head, toes touching the ground

Hanumanasana in sirsasana – the splits in headstand

Hara – the location of the soul and centre of awareness in the Zen belief system

Hare – a call to God in the omnipresent form of Vishnu

Harijan – Gandhi's name for the untouchable caste, literally 'children of god', also called *dalits*, 'the downtrodden'

Hatha yoga – a system of physical exercises and breath control

Hinduism – the Western word for India's dominant and ancient religion, known to its practitioners as *Sanatana Dharma* or the Eternal Truth. Hindus believe in one Supreme Being or *Brahman*, who is manifested in many thousands of gods and goddesses. Brahma, Shiva and Vishnu are the three principal manifestations of this Being – much like the Christian trinity of God as the Father, Son and Holy Ghost. The goal of Hinduism is liberation from the cycle of rebirth and suffering brought about by one's own actions

Hookah – tobacco pipe with a long tube that draws smoke through water

Iddly – spongy rice cake

Integral yoga – the bringing of Divine consciousness down into the yogi so that it is manifested on earth and in matter, implies a process of transformation and integration, so that the individual can stand, not alone with the demands of his ego, but in a collective soul – a new, ego-less society

Isvara – the ultimate reality; God, the Divine, or the inner guru

Isvara-pranidhana – surrendering to the ultimate reality

Iyengar yoga – style of yoga created by B.K.S. Iyengar and characterized by precise alignment and the use of props

Jai – Indian exclamation meaning praise be, offering salutations

Japa – the repetition of a mantra

Jaya – victory

Jhula – bridge

Ji – a mark of respect and reverence; for example, Guruji – most revered guru

Jiva – the personal or individual unenlightened soul, wrongly identifies itself with the mind and body

Jnana yoga – the yoga of Self-knowledge

Jnani – one who is established in the state of Self-knowledge

Kali – very fierce Hindu goddess with a bright red tongue, hair of serpents, black body and a necklace of skulls; she destroys evil spirits, protects devotees

Kapalabhati – literally 'shining skull breath' or bellows breathing

Kapha – water *dosha*, nourishes *vata* and *pitta*

Karana sharira – one of three bodies in the *Vedic* tradition, it is the location of the soul, the higher Self, pure consciousness, sometimes known as 'the Bliss Sheath'

Karma yoga – the performance of actions without attachment to results

Kathakali – a Keralan combination of dance, music and ritual in which characters with painted faces and wild costumes act out stories from Hindu epics

Keet – plaited coconut fronds, often used to make roofs

Klesha – the five causes of human affliction, mind disturbances, obstacles

Krishna – an incarnation of Vishnu, a playful cowherd, a great lover who ravished 900,000 milkmaids. Arjuna's teacher and the supreme Lord of the universe in *The Bhagavad Gita*

Kriya – cleansing technique

Kriya yoga – the practice of Svadhyaya, Tapas and Isvara-pranidhana

Ksiptam – a state of high agitation in which the mind is like a butterfly

Kumbh Mela – a Hindu festival celebrated every twelve years at four places: Haridwar; Allahabad; Ujjain; and Nasik

Kumkum – the vermilion powder that is used in puja ceremonies to anoint the forehead, said to be a representation of Devi, the Universal Mother from whom all life emanates

Kundalini – the coiled female serpent of energy; in a dormant state it lays at the base of the spine

Kurta pyjamas – trousers with matching collarless long-sleeved tunic, worn by men

Laddu – sweet deep-fried balls

Lakshmi – Hindu goddess of wealth and prosperity, Vishnu's consort

Lao Tzu – sixth-century BC Chinese philosopher, the father of Taoism

Lotus pose – *padmasana*: sitting position in which the legs are crossed and the feet rest on the opposite thighs, said to resemble the flower of the lotus

Lungi – a coloured, often checked, informal rectangular cloth worn by Indian men, usually made of cotton, tied around the waist. Often folded over to knee-length

Ma – mother

Mahamandaleshwar – the highest level of Hindu spiritual guardianship

Maharishi/Maharshi – revered spiritual teacher, sage (pronounced Marharishi)

Mala – a string of 108 meditation beads, used to help mantra repetition

Mandir – a Hindu temple

Manipura chakra – the fire *chakra*, located behind the navel

Mantra – a sacred syllable, word or phrase that helps to focus, purify and elevate the mind

Matrimandir – temple of the Mother

Meera – a female devotee in divine love with Lord Krishna

Mela – a Hindu festival

Mitra – *Vedic* god of friendship

Mudham – a dull, inert and cloudy state of mind, often associated with feelings of depression

Mudita – spiritual happiness, said to be reached through chanting, mantras and meditation

Muladhara bandha – the root or earth lock located at the base of the spine

Muladhara chakra – the root or earth chakra

Nadi – literally means 'stream', energy channel through which life force circulates in the subtle body

Namaste – traditional Indian greeting meaning 'the spirit in me respects the spirit in you'

Nandi – Shiva's bull, a symbol of fertility

Nauli – a *kriya* in which the abdominal muscles move vertically and laterally in a wave-like motion

Niyamas – the five practices that create a disciplined body and mind

Ojas Shakti – hormonal energy that creates radiance when it is transformed into higher level spiritual energy

OM – a mystical syllable incarnating the original sound of the universe, the most sacred mantra

OM Mani Padme Hum – the mantra of Chenrezig, the Buddha of Compassion

OM Namo Narayanaya – Narayanaya is a name for Vishnu, hence this mantra offers prostrations to Lord Vishnu, the preserver of the universe

Paan – betel nut, spices and limejuice in a folded leaf, chewed as a stimulant

Panchakarma – the five purifying practices that rid the body of excess *doshas* – *pitta, vata, kapha*

Paneer – milk curd cheese

Parsva pada sarvangasana – 'one-legged sideways shoulderstand pose': weight of the body is on the shoulders, one leg over the head, toes on the ground, the other leg is vertical, toes pointed

Patanjali – incarnation of Adisesha sent by Lord Vishnu to end man's suffering; he prescribed three solutions – yoga, ayurveda and Sanskrit grammar

Pitta – fire *dosha*, creates heat and light within the body

Pranava – a name used for the syllable OM; OM is known as the 'Pranava mantra'

Pranayama – practices designed to regulate the breath

Prasad – literally means 'grace', the blessed food handed out at the end of a *puja*

Prem – love

Puja – a worship ceremony

Purusha – the Eternal Self, pure consciousness

Raga – attachment, especially to pleasure

Raja – king

Raja yoga – the royal path of yoga in which the yogi seeks to become the ruler of his mind, eventually eliminating any identification with personality, in order to bring about Self-Realization. The system is codified in Patanjali's 195 sutras

Rama – hero of the epic poem 'The Ramayana', an *avatar* of Vishnu

Ramakrishna – revered religious leader who led the Hindu renaissance in the nineteenth century

Rishi – a sage or seer of truth to whom the wisdom of the *Vedas* was revealed

Sadhu – a holy person, a renunciate who lives the age-old ideals of the eremitical life, has no fixed abode

Sahasra padma chakra – located at the crown, it has 1,000 petals and is the seat of consciousness

Saivite – worshipper of Shiva

Salwar kameez – long tunic and loose trousers worn by women

Samadhi – the ultimate state of yoga, enlightenment itself, a state of intense concentration and sublime peace in which the yogi can see the object of his meditation without distortion and is in union with universal consciousness or the Supreme spirit – like a drop of water in the ocean

Samkalpa – hopes, expectations, intentions, will and motivation; the mental action used to create *samskaras*

Samskara – the habits and subconscious conditionings of the mind

Samyoga – union

Sanga – a group of like-minded seekers

Sanskrit – the ancient language of India, the Indian equivalent of Latin

Santoor – traditional Indian instrument, a 'one-hundred-stringed lute'

Santosha – contentment

Saraswati – Brahma's consort, goddess of learning and wisdom

Sarvangasana – 'shoulderstand': the head and shoulders are on the floor, the lower body and legs are supported by the hands and point straight up in the air

Sat – permanent reality, being, truth, existence

Sat-chit-ananda – existence-consciousness-bliss, the essence of Brahman

Satsang – a group of truth-seekers

Sattvic – pure, harmonious, serene, in balance; one of three *gunas* or qualities of nature

Satya – truthfulness

Saucha – purity of mind and body

Savasana – 'corpse pose': final relaxation at the end of a yoga practice

Savitri – Hindu goddess, daughter of the sun; also Sri Aurobindo's epic poem

Shakti – Shiva's consort, the female creative force in the universe

Shala – yoga practice place

Shanti – peace

Shiva – one of the trinity of Hindu gods, Shiva is the destroyer who lived in the Himalaya or Varanasi, the Lord of Yoga

Shiva linga – one of the forms in which Shiva is worshipped. A *yin-yang* symbol portraying the eternal embrace of cosmic masculine and feminine higher forces and creative power

Sirsasana – headstand

Sitar – a large, long-necked Indian lute

Sivananda yoga – a system of yoga drawn from the *Hatha* and *Raja* traditions. The system was created by Swami Vishnu-devananda, founder of the Sivananda Yoga Vedanta centres and a disciple of Sivananda, the Hindu founder of the Divine Life mission

Somatics – exercises developed by Thomas Hanna, a disciple of Feldenkrais, designed to bring awareness to the body

Sri (also Shri) – Indian title of respect; honourable, holy

Sthiram – stability, alertness and attention

Sthula sharira – one of three bodies in the *Vedic* tradition; the physical body

Sukha(m) – lightness, feeling at ease, comfortable

Sukshma sharira – one of three bodies in the *Vedic* tradition; the astral body

Supramental Consciousness – truth consciousness, necessary for the transformation of terrestrial life into Divine life

Sushumna – the main energy channel running up the centre of the astral spine, the most significant *nadi*

Sutra – literally 'thread', the yoga sutras are aphorisms on yoga

Svadhyaya – the study of spiritual literature

Svadishthana chakra – the water or sex *chakra*

Swami – a monk, a Self-Realized teacher, a master of the Self

Tablas – a pair of Indian hand drums

Tantra yoga – rejects the *Vedic* idea that *samadhi* is only attainable through asceticism. *Tantrics* believe that the body is a temple of the Divine, and a means for achieving *samadhi*. The so-called 'right-handed path' is highly disciplined, insisting on purity of thought and action; the 'left-handed path' (for example, Osho) is more liberal, allowing sexual practices in the pursuit of spiritual ecstasy

Tapas – 'that which generates heat', purifying acts that increase spiritual fervour

Tara – a female Buddha, associated with compassion, rescues beings from suffering

Tat Sat – that which I am, I am That

Thali – Indian compartmentalized plate offering a selection of food

Tilaka – a ritual mark on the forehead, said to cool the spot between the eyebrows, traditionally the seat of wisdom and concentration, as an aid to meditation and the merging of Atman with Brahman. Specific markings denote sectarian allegiances

Tittibhasana – 'firefly pose': balancing on the hands, legs pointing forward around the outer arms, toes pointed, looking forwards

Transcendental Meditation – the mind transcends all mental activity to experience the simplest form of awareness, so-called Transcendental Consciousness. Its practice is said to send out harmonic vibes for world peace

Tundu – wide headband

Uddiyana bandha – abdominal lock

Uttanasana – 'standing forward fold': a standing position in which the forehead is brought down and in, towards the shins

Utthita hasta padangusthasana – 'extended hand to big toe posture': balancing on one leg, the opposite leg is extended in front, the big toe held in the hand

Vairagya – renunciation

Vaishnavite – worshipper of Vishnu

Vata – wind *dosha*, creates energy, life, movement in the body

Vedas – literally means 'knowledge', the oldest sacred Hindu texts (3,500 BC), yoga first defined here as 'yoking'

Veena – a seven-stringed musical instrument

Veshti – a formal version of a *dhoti*, a veshti with a gold embroidered border is often seen at ceremonies, worn with a white shirt

Vibhuti – sacred grey ash that Shiva smeared on himself, now practised by many *sadhus*, believed to restore the dead to life

Vinyasa – literally a 'special arrangement', denotes a particular sequence of postures

Vipassana – literally 'insight' or 'clear seeing', a meditation that watches the body and its sensations.

Virabhadrasana I – 'warrior I': one leg stretched straight out 3 or 4 feet behind, toes pointing to 45 degrees, other leg bent deeply to 90 degrees, both arms above head, facing forward

Virabhadrasana II – 'warrior II': one leg stretched straight out 3 or 4 feet behind, toes pointing to 45 degrees, other leg bent deeply to 90 degrees, arms and torso rotated to 180 degrees

Virasana – 'hero's pose', sitting between the heels with thigh bones parallel

Vishnu – one of the trinity of Hindu gods, Vishnu is the preserver of the universe, appears in ten *avatars* including Krishna and Rama

Vishuddha chakra – the ether *chakra*, located at the throat

Vivek – insight, wisdom

Vritti – thoughts which prevent the seeing of truth

Yamas – the five moral codes of conduct that govern how we behave to other people in our daily life

Yin-Yang – symbolizing the duality of life in which neither quality can exist without the other. Yin is passive, female, water; Yang is active, male, fire

Yoga – from *'yuj'* meaning 'to join' or 'yoke', to bring together into union, the union of mind, body, breath and spirit, and the union between individual consciousness and the universal consciousness, the disciplined science of Self-Realization in which the mind is focused, one-pointedness developed and *samadhi* experienced

Yogi – a follower of the discipline of yoga

Zen – a Japanese school of Buddhism

Useful Contacts

UK

Iyengar Institute

223 Randolph Avenue, London W9 1NL

www.iyi.org.uk • 0207 624 3080

Free Spirit Travel – yoga holiday specialists

153 Carden Avenue, Brighton BN1 8LA

www.freespirituk.com • info@freespirituk.com • 01273 564 230

The Life Centre

15 Edge Street, London W8 7PN

For information about classes, holidays & teacher training: www.thelifecentre.com

General enquiries: info@thelifecentre.com

Teacher training enquiries: teachertraining@thelifecentre.com • 0207 221 4602

Simon Low

For information about yoga holidays, residential weekends and classes:

www.simonlow.com • Teacher training: www.theyogaacademy.org

For all enquiries: 0207 722 1682

Sivananda Yoga Centre

51 Felsham Road, London SW15 1AZ

www.sivananda.org/london • london@sivananda.org • 0208 780 0160

Triyoga

Primrose Hill: 6 Erskine Road, London NW3 3AJ

Covent Garden: Neal's Yard Therapy Rooms, 2 Neal's Yard, London WC2

www.triyoga.co.uk • For all enquiries: 0207 483 3344

INDIA

GOA

The Purple Valley Yoga Centre

www.yogagoa.net

KARNATAKA (MYSORE – PATTABHI JOIS, MR VENKATESH)

Sri K. Pattabhi Jois

Ashtanga Yoga Research Institute, #235 8th Cross, 3rd Stage, Gokulam,

Mysore 570002, Karnataka

www.ayri.org • +91 821 251 6756

Mr Venkatesh

Atma Vikasa Centre of Yogic Sciences, Exactly opp. Nalpak Resturant,

Kuvempunagar Double Road, Mysore 570009, Karnataka

www.atmavikasa.com • atmavikasa@eth.net • +91 821 234 1978

KERALA (AMMA, SIVANANDA)

Amma

Mata Amritanandamayi Math, Amritapuri P.O. Kollam Dist., Kerala 690525

www.amritapuri.org • inform@amritapuri.org • +91 476 289 6399/7578/6278

Sivananda Yoga Vedanta Dhanwantari Ashram

P.O. Neyyar Dam, Thiruvananthapuram 695572, Kerala

www.sivananda.org/ndam • yogaindia@sivananda.org • +91 471 227 3093

MAHARASHTRA (PUNE – B.K.S. IYENGAR, OSHO)

B.K.S. Iyengar

Ramamani Iyengar Memorial Yoga Institute, 1107 B/1 Hare Krishna Mandir
Road, Model Colony, Shivaji Nagar, Pune – 411015, Maharashtra
Contact Mr Pandurang Rao (Secretary)
www.bksiyengar.com • +91 202 565 6134

Osho

Osho International Resort, 17 Koregaon Park, Pune MS 411001, Maharashtra
+91 20 401 9999 • www.osho.com • resortinfo@osho.net
For the guesthouse: www.osho.com/resort/guesthouse • reservations@osho.com

TAMIL NADU (AUROVILLE, T.K.V. DESIKACHAR, RAMANA MAHARSHI)

Afsanah's

Afsanah's Guesthouse, Kottakarai, Auroville 605111, T.C. Balam, Tamil Nadu
www.afsanah.com • afsanah_gh@auroville.org.in • +91 413 2622 108

Aurobindo Ashram

Sri Aurobindo's Ashram, Bureau Central, Information Centre of Sri Aurobindo
Ashram, Cottage Complex, 3 Rangapillai Street, Pondicherry 605001, Tamil Nadu
www.sriaurobindoashram.org • bureaucentral@sriaurobindoashram.org
+91 413 339 648

Auroville

Auroville Universal Township Secretariat, Bharat Nivas, Auroville 605101,
Tamil Nadu
www.auroville.org • info@auroville.org.in

T.K.V. Desikachar

Krishnamacharya Yoga Mandiram, 31, Fourth Cross Street, R K Nagar,
Chennai 600 028, Tamil Nadu
www.kym.org • studies@kym.org • +91 44 2493 3092/246 20202

Down's Syndrome Association of Tamil Nadu

For more information contact:

Mrs Rekha Ramachandran, Mathru Mandir Down's Syndrome of Tamil Nadu, 50 Sriman Srinivasan Road, Alwarpet, Chennai 600 018

mathrumandir@vsnl.net • +91 44 2498 6824

Ideal Beach Resort

Ideal Beach Resort, Mahabalipuram – 603 104, Tamil Nadu

www.idealresort.com • +91 4114 242240/242443/243043

New Woodlands Hotel

New Woodlands Hotel, 72-75 Dr.Radhakrishnan Road, P.B No 626, Mylapore, Chennai 600004, Tamil Nadu

www.newwoodlands.com • reserve@newwoodlands.com • +91 44 2811 3111

Ramana Maharshi

Sri Ramanasramam, Tiruvannamali, Tamil Nadu 606 603

www.ramana-maharshi.org • ashram@ramana-maharshi.org

+91 4175 237 292/237 200

Address all communications to The President

UTTARANCHAL (RISHIKESH – DIVINE LIFE SOCIETY, VINAY P. MENON, PANKASH, PRIMOD, SHANTIMAYI)

Ananda in the Himalayas

The Palace Estate, Narendra Nagar, Tehri Garhwal, Uttaranchal 249175

www.anandaspa.com • sales@anandaspa.com • +91 1378 227 500

Ma Anandamayee

To book accommodation at the International Centre next door (you can't stay at the ashram) contact the manager Dr S.K. Ghosh (the address is as per the ashram): Shree Shree Ma Anandamayee Ashram Daksh Mandir Road, P.O. Kankhal, Distt. Hardwar (U.R) 249408

www.anandamayi.org

Rudra Dev

The Yoga Study Centre, Ganga Vihar, Haridwar Road, Rishikesh 249201

+91 135 431 196.

Divine Life Society

Write to The General Secretary stating why you want to visit and how long for.

NB: When writing for the first time the maximum stay is likely to be one week/ten days.

PO Sivananda Nagar 249192, Distt. Tehri Garhwal, Uttaranchal, Himalaya

www.divinelifesociety.org

The Great Ganga Hotel

Muni-Ki-Reti, Rishikesh 249 201, Uttaranchal

www.thegreatganga.com • hotelthegreatganga@yahoo.co.in • +91 135 244 2243

Jaipur Gems Centre

Lakshman Jhula, Rishikesh 249 302, Uttaranchal • +91 135 243 1255

Madras Café

Shivanand Nagar, Tehri Garhwal, Uttaranchal 249 201 • +91 135 243 3219

Vinay and Lavenya Menon – now in Dubai at the Six Senses Spa

Six Senses Spa, Madinat Jumeirah – the Arabian Resort, PO Box 75157

Dubai, United Arab Emirates

www.madinatjumeirah.com • www.sixsenses.com • +971 4 3668888

Pankash

The Green Hotel, Swargashram

Primod

The Yoga Hut, By 1st auto rickshaw stand, Tapovan Sarai,

West Lakshman Jhula Bridge

Yoga_instructor@indiatimes.com • +91 135 243 6842

Sadhana Mandir Trust (Swami Rama's original ashram)

Ramnagar, P.O. Pashulok, Rishikesh 249 203, Uttaranchal

sadhanamandir@vsnl.com • +91 135 431 485/435 799/431 693

ShantiMayi

Sacha Dham Ashram, Laxman Jhula, P.O. Tapovan Sarai 249192, Tehri Garhwal
Uttaranchal

www.shantimayi.com • omguru2001@yahoo.com • + 91 135 433 184

Sivananda Emporium Bookshop (yoga and astrology)

Swargashram 249 304, Uttaranchal

+91 135 243 2795

Sonu (owner of great music shop)

Kala Sangam Studio, Ram Jhula, Near taxi stand, opp. Madras Café, Rishikesh,
Uttaranchal

+91 135 243 4779

Swami Rama Sadhaka Grama (Swami Veda's new ashram)

Vill. Virpur Khurd, Virbhadra Road, Rishikesh, Uttaranchal 249 203

srsg@vsnl.com • +91 135 450 093/453 030/452 978/79

Triveni Travel Services

Buta Ram MD, Haridwar Road, Rishikesh, Uttaranchal

triveni_travels@rediffmail.com • 0135 243 0989

TURKEY

Huzur Vadisi

Gokceovacik, Gocek 48310, Fethiye

www.huzurvadisi.com • + 90 252 644 0008

Further Reading

India

Brown, Mick, *The Spiritual Tourist* (London: Bloomsbury, 1998)

Brunton, Paul, *A Search in Secret India* (London: Rider, 2003)

Dalrymple, William, *City of Djinns* (London: Flamingo, 1994), *The Age of Kali* (London: Flamingo, 1999)

Macdonald, Sarah, *Holy Cow – An Indian Adventure* (Australia: Bantam, 2002)

Mehta, Gita, *Karma Cola* (India: Penguin, 1993)

Guide to the yogis, gurus and ashrams of India

Cushman, Anne and Jerry Jones, *From Here to Nirvana* (London: Rider, 1998)

Yoga theory and practice

Cope, Stephen, *Yoga and the Quest for the True Self* (New York: Bantam, 1999)

Davis, Jeff, *The Journey From the Center to the Page – Yoga Philosophies and Practices as Muse for Authentic Writing* (New York: Penguin, 2004)

Desikachar, T.K.V., *The Heart of Yoga* (Rochester: Inner Traditions, 1995), *Reflections on Yoga Sutras of Patanjali* (India: KYM Publications, 2003)

Farhi, Donna, *Bringing Yoga to Life* (New York: HarperCollins, 2003)

Feuerstein, Georg, *The Deeper Dimension of Yoga* (Boston: Shambhala Publications, 2003)

Gannon, Sharon and David Life, *Jivamukti Yoga* (New York: Ballantine, 2002)

Godman, David, ed., *Be As You Are – The Teachings of Sri Ramana Maharshi* (India: Penguin, 1992)

Iyengar, B.K.S., *Light on Yoga* (India: HarperCollins, 2000)

Jois, Sri K. Pattabhi, *Yoga Mala* (New York: Eddie Stern/Patanjali Yoga Shala, 2000)

Krishna, Gopala, *The Yogi – Portraits of Swami Vishnu-devananda* (India: New Age Books, 2002)

Mascaro, Juan, transl., *The Bhagavad Gita* (London: Penguin, 1962)

Osho, *Autobiography of a Spiritually Incorrect Mystic* (New York: St Martins Press, 2001), *From Sex to Superconsciousness* (India: Full Circle Publishing, 2003)

Pandit, M.P., *Dictionary of Sri Aurobindo's Yoga* (India: Dipti Publications, 1973)

Saltzman, Paul, *The Beatles in Rishikesh* (New York: Viking Studio, PenguinPutnam, 2000)

Schiffman, Erich, *Yoga – The Spirit and Practice of Moving Into Stillness* (New York: Pocket Books, 1996)

Sparrowe, Linda, *Yoga* (A *Yoga Journal* book, 2002)

Vishnu-devananda, Swami, *Meditation and Mantras* (India: Motilal Banarsidass Publishers, 2001)

Yogananda, Paramahansa, *Autobiography of a Yogi* (London: Rider, 1996)

Permissions

Extract from *Auroville Architecture, Towards New Forms For a New Consciousness* by kind permission of PRISMA at Auroville (prisma@auroville.org.in).

Extract from *The Matrimandir* by kind permission of Matrimandir, Auroville (auroville.org.in).

Chants and extracts from the *Atma Vikasa Instructions for Students* by kind permission of Atma Vikasa Centre of Yogic Sciences (www.atmavikasa.com).

Permission to publish the *'Jaya Ganesha'* chant from the *Sivananda Yoga Vedanta Satsang Chant Book* kindly given by the Sivananda Yoga Vedanta Centre (www.sivananda.org/london).

Permission to quote from *Reflections on Yoga Sutra-s of Patanjali* by Shri T.K.V. Desikachar kindly given by the publisher Krishnamacharya Yoga Mandiram (www.kym.org).

Permission to quote from *Shri T. Krishnamacharya – The Legend Lives On* kindly given by the publisher Krishnamacharya Yoga Mandiram.

Permission to quote extracts from *The Yogi – Portraits of Swami Vishnu-devananda* by Gopala Krishna kindly given by the publisher Yes International Publishers of USA (www.yespublishers.com).

Extract from *A Search in Secret India* by Paul Brunton published by Rider. Used by kind permission of The Random House Group Limited (www.randomhouse.co.uk).

Extract from *The Song of the Poppadam* by Ramana Maharshi appears in *The Collected Works of Ramana Maharshi*, edited by Arthur Osborne and published by Sri Ramanasramam. Used by kind permission of the president, Sri Ramanasramam, Tiruvannamalai. (www.ramana-maharshi.org).

Extract from *Sri Maharshi A Short Life Sketch*, published by Sri Ramanasramam. Used by kind permission of the president, Sri Ramanasramam, Tiruvannamalai.

Extracts from *Be As You Are, The Teachings of Sri Ramana Maharshi* by David Godman, published by Penguin. Used by kind permission of the president, Sri Ramanasramam, Tiruvannamalai.

Extracts from *Dictionary of Sri Aurobindo's Yoga* by M.P. Pandit, published by Dipti Publications, Sri Aurobindo Ashram, Pondicherry, reprinted with the kind permission of the Sri Aurobindo Ashram Trust. (www.sriaurobindoashram.org).

Extract from *The Big Blue* with the kind permission of Société Gaumont, France (www.gaumont.fr).

Thanks

This book would not have been written without my writing gurus, Chris Stewart and Ian Marchant, to whom I owe a river of alcohol. They read the early material, handed over the names of their publishers and agents with wild abandon and told me, quite firmly in fact, that I could do it.

Annette Green and David Smith are awesome agents whose reckless enthusiasm for the book met its match at Ebury in the form of my equally awesome editor Hannah MacDonald, her assistant editor Claire Kingston, Caroline Newbury in Publicity, Dawn Burnett in Marketing, and Ken Barlow who did just about everything else.

Thanks to all of my family. To Dad for giving Lucy in the Sky with Diamonds a love of books and adventure – reading me stories about far away lands in which curious children explored treacherous terrains, hidden underground passages and mysterious castles on the hill, children who acted heroically, and always got back in time for tea. To Mum for her gleeful observation and wit, for giving up her workroom to the cause, roadtesting muffins, making me endless ham sandwiches and rubbing my aching neck. To Oliver for selflessly tasting the muffins, reading everything and not being too liberal with his red pen. To Nikki for religiously keeping the pink files in order. To Toria and Jo, Tom and Jo, Matthew, Aunty Phyllis and Hilda for their unquestioning encouragement, and to Teddy for his luminous smile.

Simon Low gave me a life-changing introduction to yoga, helped me peel back the layers of the onion and was there with a box of tissues when it all got too much. Jen Norman, a true Yoga Goddess, continued the work and held me tight whenever I wobbled.

Thanks to the Cappuccino Gurus – Paola de Carolis, Natasha Harvey, Pia Jones, Danielle Roffe – who believed in me, and were endlessly patient in my hours of angst.

Norman Blair, Graham Burns, Daniel Cook, Paola de Carolis, Jen and Jeff Phenix and Pia Jones read through the first ramblings, were honest and constructive in their criticism and didn't snigger – at least not in front of me.

Thanks to all of the people who read my long emails home and encouraged me to put my ramblings into a book – many of those mentioned above, plus Magnus Blair, Mark Bridgeford, Nik Elsome, Matt Fone, Nigel Gilderson, Andy Glynn, Sophie Grenville, Ruth Hassall, Sarah Hatherley, Wrenne Hiscott, Anna Hughes, Clare Hutchinson, Susan Lynch, Nicky May, John McDonald, Gareth Miles, Princess Cassie Moore, Christophe Mouze, Jenifer Otwell, Clare Roberts, Katie Sutton, Miles and Louise Taylor, Rosie Walford and Lawrence Webb.

Thanks to the yoga students I met along the way who made dropping out so much more fun – Maria Lusia Marcadar Albert, Runa Basu, Sarah Batho, Leif Bremark, Reid Bruggemann, Annabel Chown, Linda Cope, Jeff Davis, Michael Dinuri, Chris Drynan, Sharon Elias, Egil Eriksen, Dermot Feenan, Bruce Goodison, Marion Gourlay, Emma Henry, Tracy Jeune, Gaultier Lechelle, Tiffany Lee, Sara Moloney, Pia Muggerud, Sachiyo Munechika, Matt Nash, Christine Nystrup, Wendy Pryke, Irene and Scott Sadler, Marta Salonidou, Christine

Schlenker, Daniel Sharon, Cory Smith, Anna Tjarnberg, Mollie Tribell, Otto Vogt, Jude Warren, Masako Yamano, and to Simon Lambert – never a yoga student but brilliant nonetheless.

Thank you to the founder members of the Ladies' Society – Alison Glynn, Maria Glynn, Heather McColm, Ness Merritt, Kerst Morris, Liz Walker – for sending me off and welcoming me home with so many bottles of Pinot Grigio.

Thanks to Graham Burns, Elizabeth Stanley and Frances Ruffelle for their generous hospitality and for not showing their concern at the size of my suitcases when I arrived on their doorsteps.

Thanks to everyone involved in the Arvon Foundation's Travel Writing course at Totleigh Barton, May 2003 – especially the lovely Janet Hodgson, and our tutors Dea Birkett and Paul Hyland.

Much respect to the Society of Authors for their expert guidance through the thorny bushes of permissions and contracts, and to Kara May for her support on the walks and at the parties!

Thanks to Kevin Wood for building the website with such love and enthusiasm.

Love and thanks to all the 'ordinary' people I met in India – especially Mahipal Singh Bisht, Vinay and Lavenya Menon, Gabriel von Radloff, Swami Shiva Swaroopananda, the teachers and students of the Krishnamacharya Yoga Mandiram, and to Goupi – through your grace I am now convinced that a merger with cosmic bliss is a definite possibility, though perhaps not in this lifetime.

And finally thank you to all the yoga students around the world. I look forward to practising next to you one day – as Henri would say: 'Atcha! OM! Boom!'